Color Your Way Through Anxiety

35 Unique, Full Page Patterns and

Words of Encouragement for Anxiety Sufferers

By Nerine Martin

ColorYourWayToHappy.com

Free

While you wait for 'Color Your Way Through Anxiety' Adult Coloring Book to arrive...... pop on over to **www.ColorYourWayToHappy.com/Freebie** and subscribe to the weekly newsletter and you will receive a FREE coloring book to print at home!

OTHER COLORING BOOKS BY NERINE MARTIN

Mandalas for Mindfulness Volume 1
Mandalas for Mindfulness Volume 2
Neon Mandalas for Mindfulness Volume 3
Patterns for Mindfulness: RELAX
My Coloring Organizer

You can also find Nerine's designs in:
Adult Coloring Book Treasury 1
Adult Coloring Book Treasury 2

Available from Amazon.com (search for Nerine Martin)
Digital versions are available for instant download from www.ColorYourWayToHappy.com

Cover and Book Design by Nerine Martin

Copyright © 2016 Nerine Martin. All rights reserved.

www.ColorYourWayToHappy.com

No part of this book may be reproduced, copied or scanned except for your own personal use and enjoyment. You may share only the images that you have colored on social media, as long as you attribute Nerine Martin and include the book name in your post.
These images, either colored or non-colored may not be resold.

ISBN: 978-1537564654

A message from the Artist.....

Congratulations on your purchase of *'Color Your Way Through Anxiety'* and thank you for choosing my coloring book.

As a keen crafter, scrap-booker, coloring enthusiast and Military Veteran, I have personally designed each page with the focus of helping other Military Veterans, and Men and Women living with conditions such as stress, anxiety & depression.

It has been proven that using coloring as a form of art therapy, can help relieve symptoms by distracting the mind's thought processes and can also aid as a coping strategy to get through those difficult times, such as a panic attack.

Inside this coloring book you will find 35 unique, full page patterns, one to color every day of the month. The pages are printed with a pattern design on one side only with words of encouragement to focus on while you color.

Use your imagination to make these patterns come alive with color, using colored pencils, felt tip markers, gel pens, fluoro markers, metallic pens or crayons. To help prevent any bleed through when using felt tip markers – place a blank sheet of paper behind the page when coloring. You can find spare pages located at the back of this book.

Please remember that your purchase of this coloring book is for your personal use only and you may not share or copy the uncolored pages for others. Please direct other people to purchase their own copy. By doing so, you are supporting my art so I can continue to make more coloring books and I thank you for your understanding and support. ☺

I have also included some bonus illustrations at the back of this book, which are a sample of designs from my mindfulness series of coloring books published so far.

I truly hope these words of encouragement can make a difference to how you are thinking and feeling, and that they can bring some calm to your life as you color them. My wish is to help other people just like you, through my coloring books, so that YOU are in total control of your life, not the anxiety!

As a long term anxiety sufferer, I know first-hand what it's like to experience anxiety and panic attacks on a daily basis. Since using coloring as part of my therapy, I have become more aware of my thoughts and now challenge them rather than let them take control. I continue to color every day and also practice mindfulness skills. This has made a big difference to my quality of life and my family's.

I wish you all the best and hope you enjoy 'Color Your Way Through Anxiety'.

Nerine ☺

P.S. If you enjoy this book, please leave a review on Amazon.

What customers have to say about the 'COLOR YOUR WAY TO HAPPY' series of Adult Coloring Books........

"Your mandalas are the most beautiful I've seen anywhere and super gorgeous with the black backgrounds. I want to encourage everyone in this group to order a copy…..
Nerine's designs are different from any others you've seen, and they are featured in Adult Coloring Book Treasury 1 and 2" – Shela W.

"I got the mandala volume one and am having a ball with it.
Mandala addicts like me, it is a must have" – Nessa

"Thank you for drawing beautiful pieces that I can put color to.
Coloring is my sanity, your pieces are calming and relaxing to color" – Christina

"Just Wonderful. Love this book! Can spend hours losing yourself in the mandala designs! Very calming and a great way to de-stress!" – Natalatalie

"…I love the story about this artist and why she did this series of books" – PINPOP

"I'm really enjoying volume 1..." – Emma

"I received these yesterday and OMG they're beyond awesome!!! Thank you heaps…" – Chelle

"Thank you for creating such an awesome coloring book with black backgrounds.
They are my favorite!" – Shela

"Beautiful Mandalas! If you just love mandalas, or want to distress this book will help with that. I love this series of coloring book each one is different in the presentation of the mandalas" – PINPOP

"One Mandala a day – great idea!" - Shelly

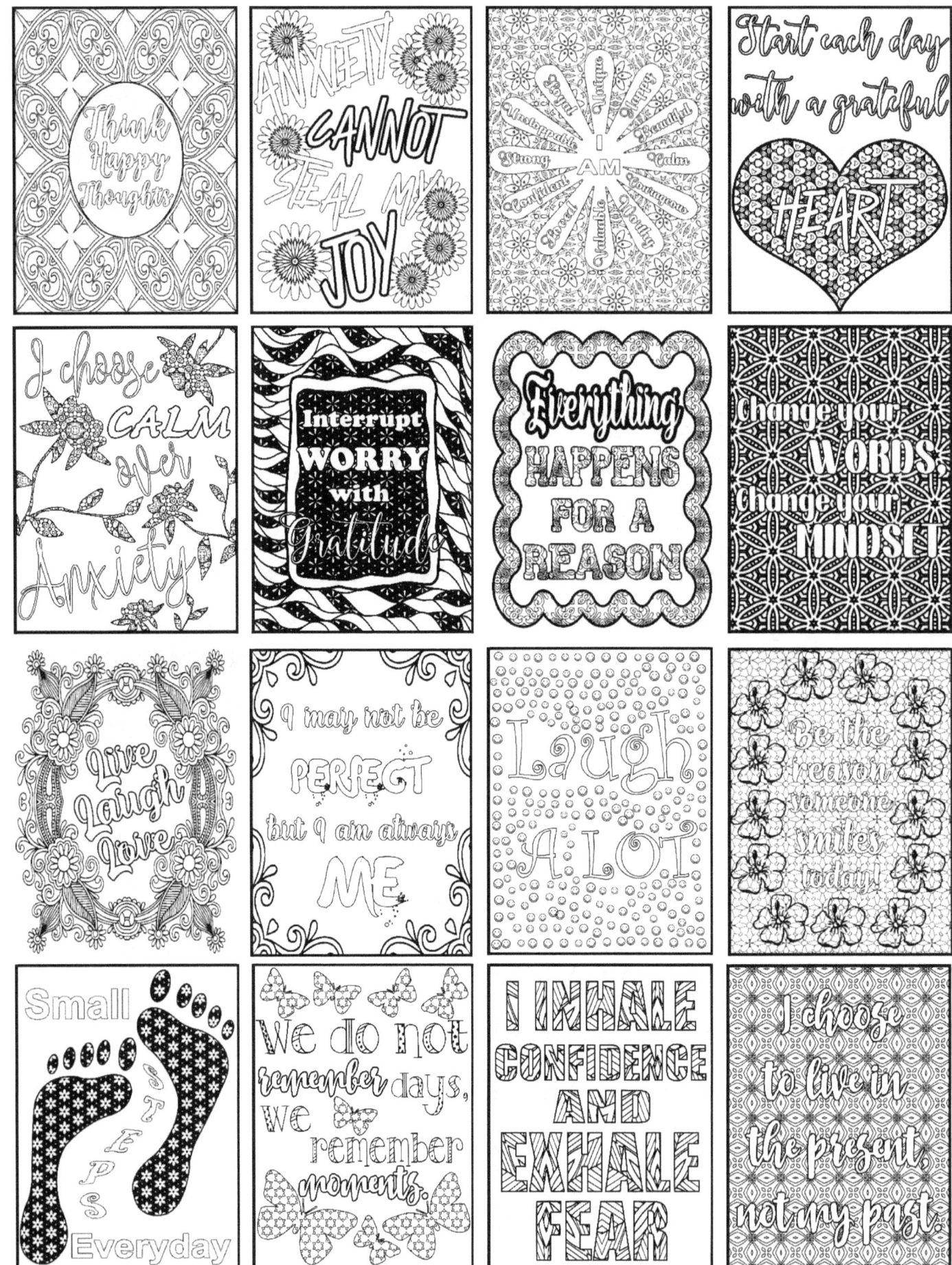

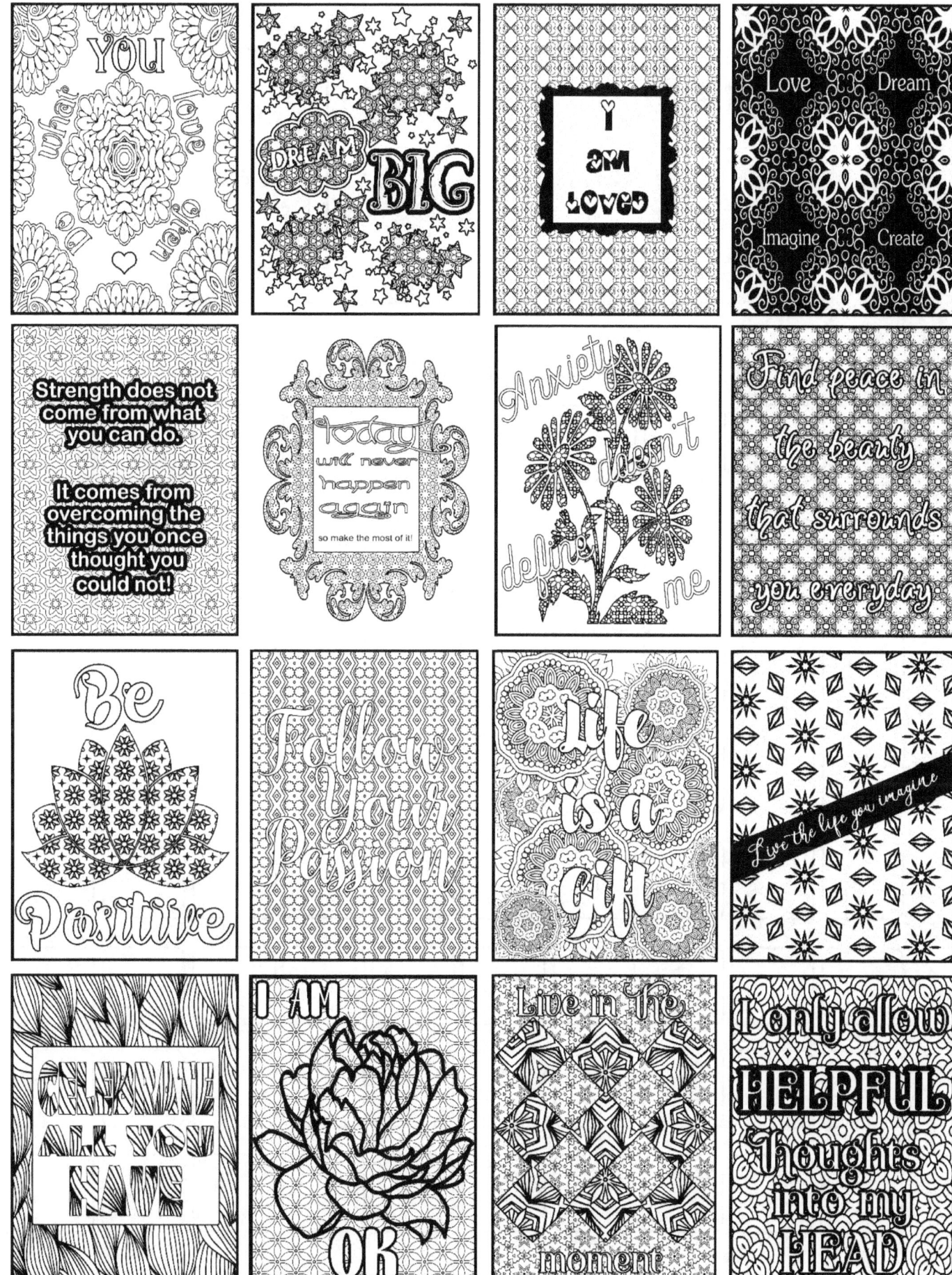

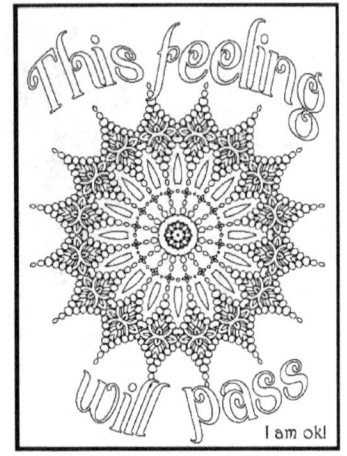 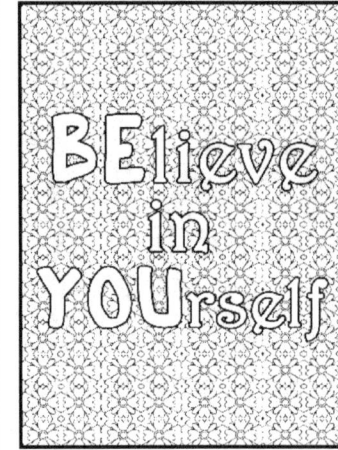 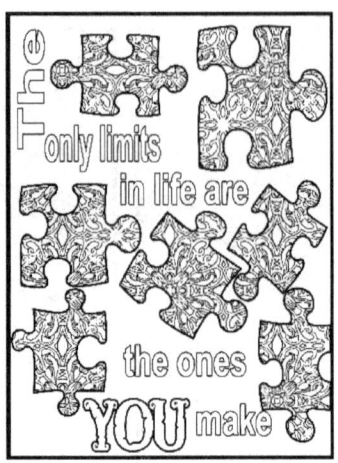

Use This Area To Test Your Colors

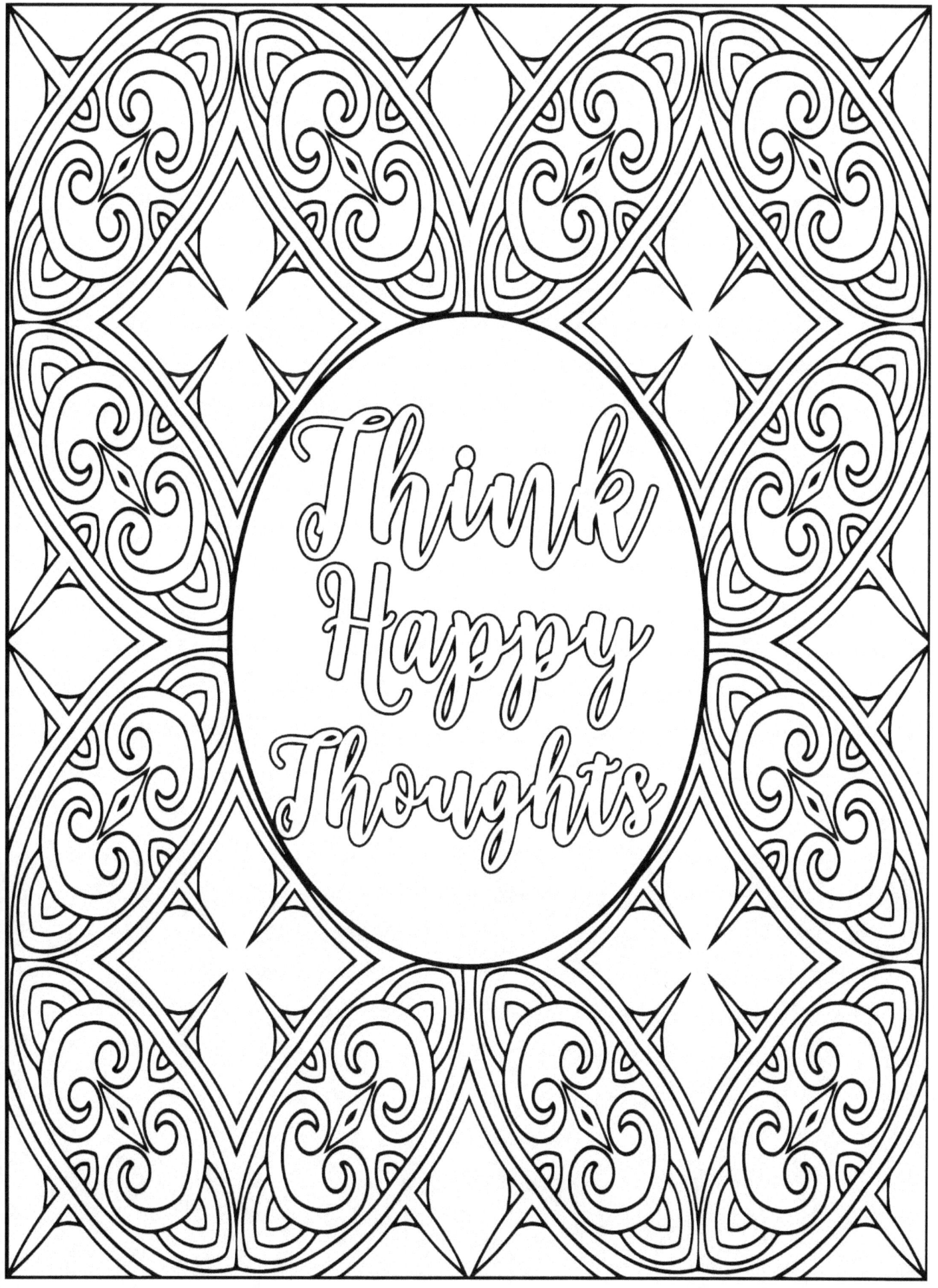

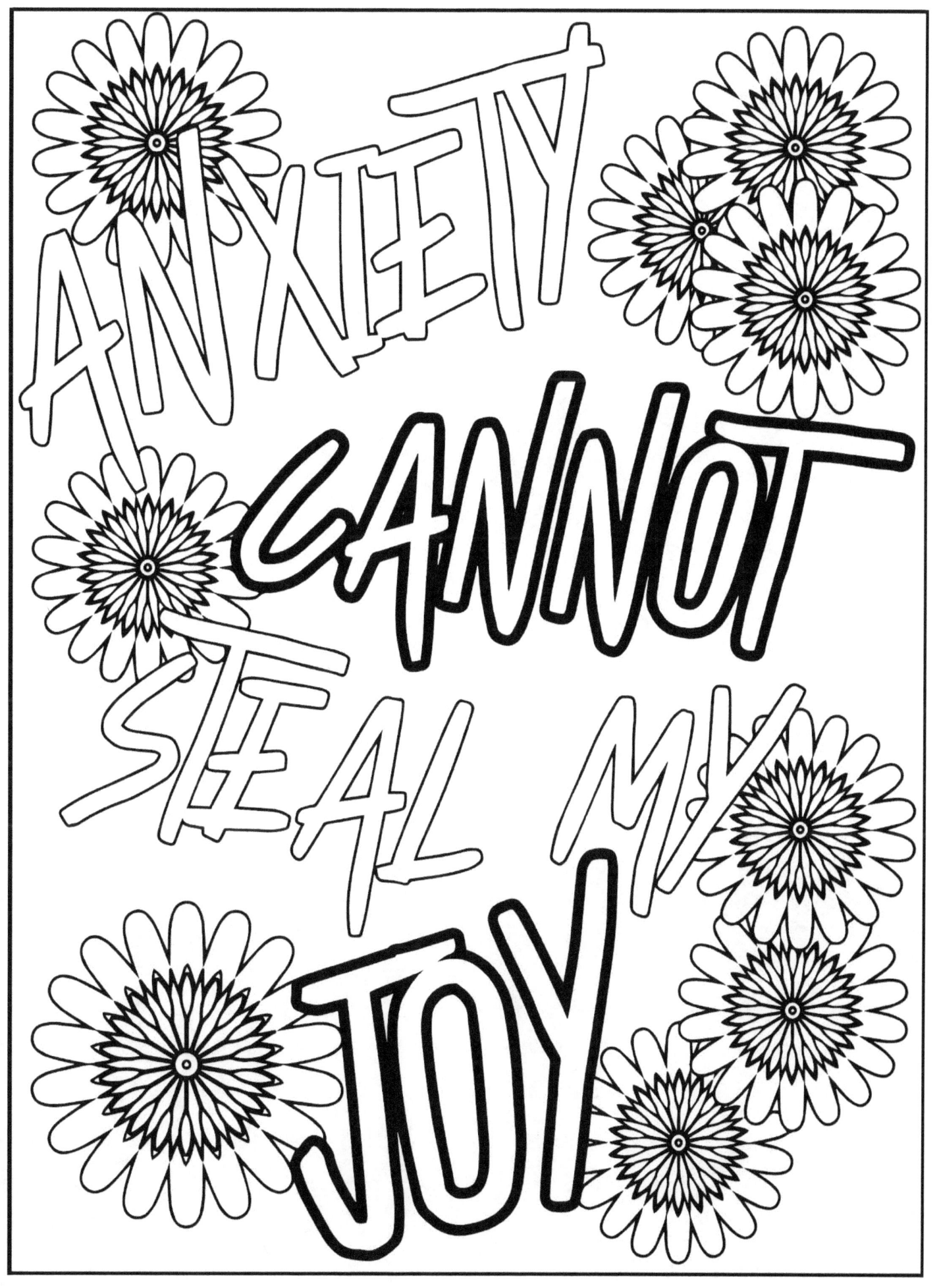

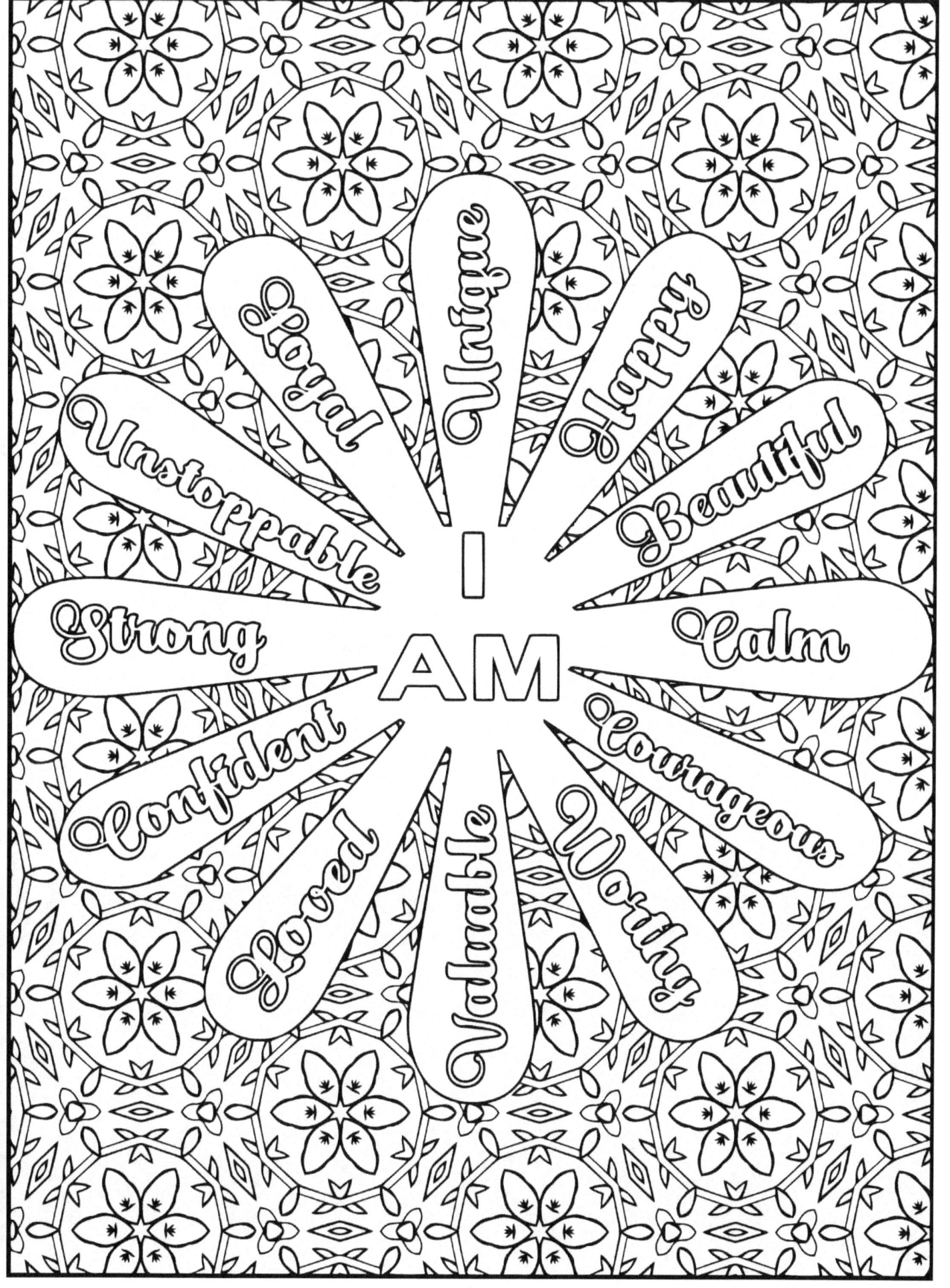

Start each day with a grateful HEART

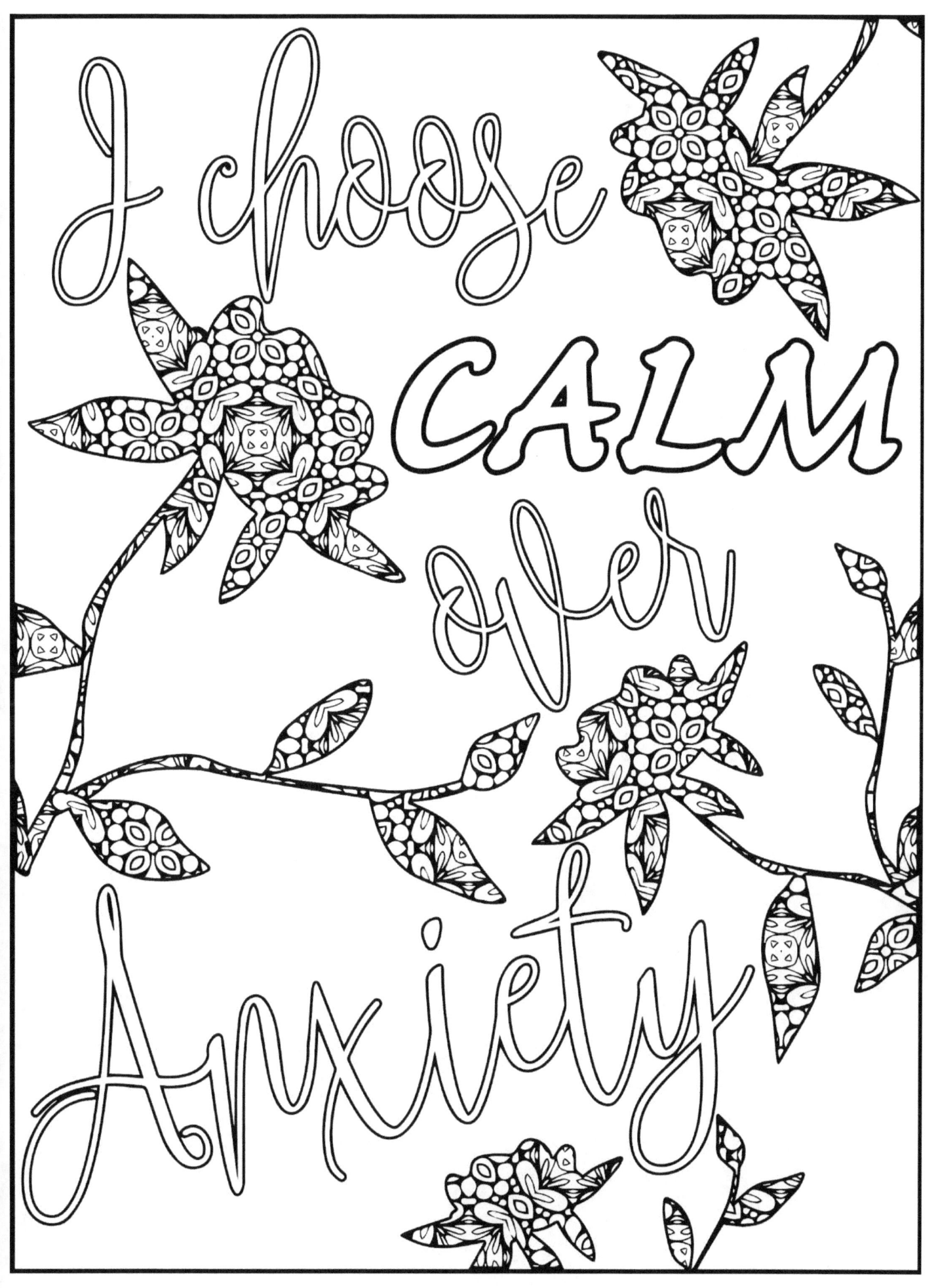

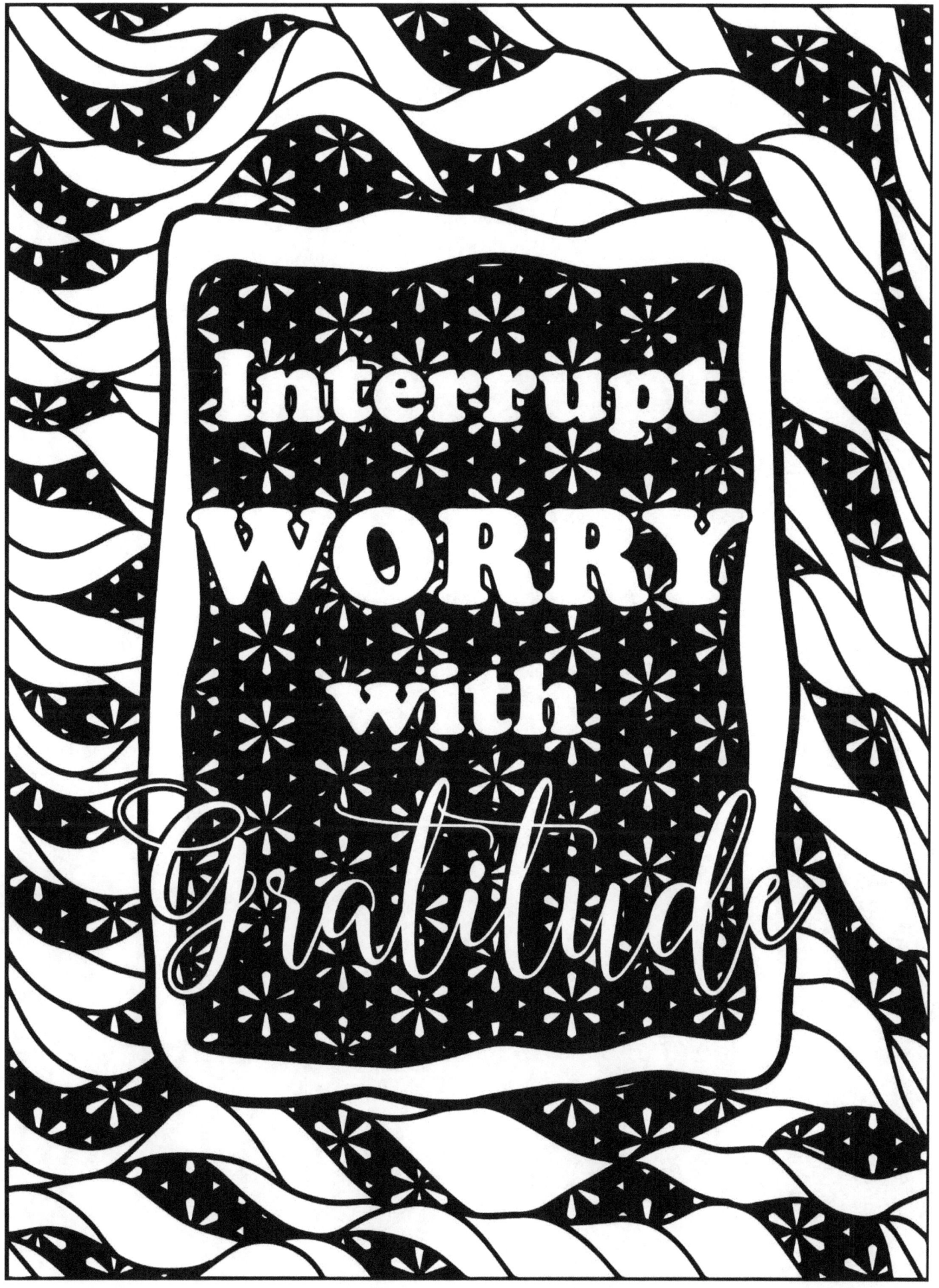

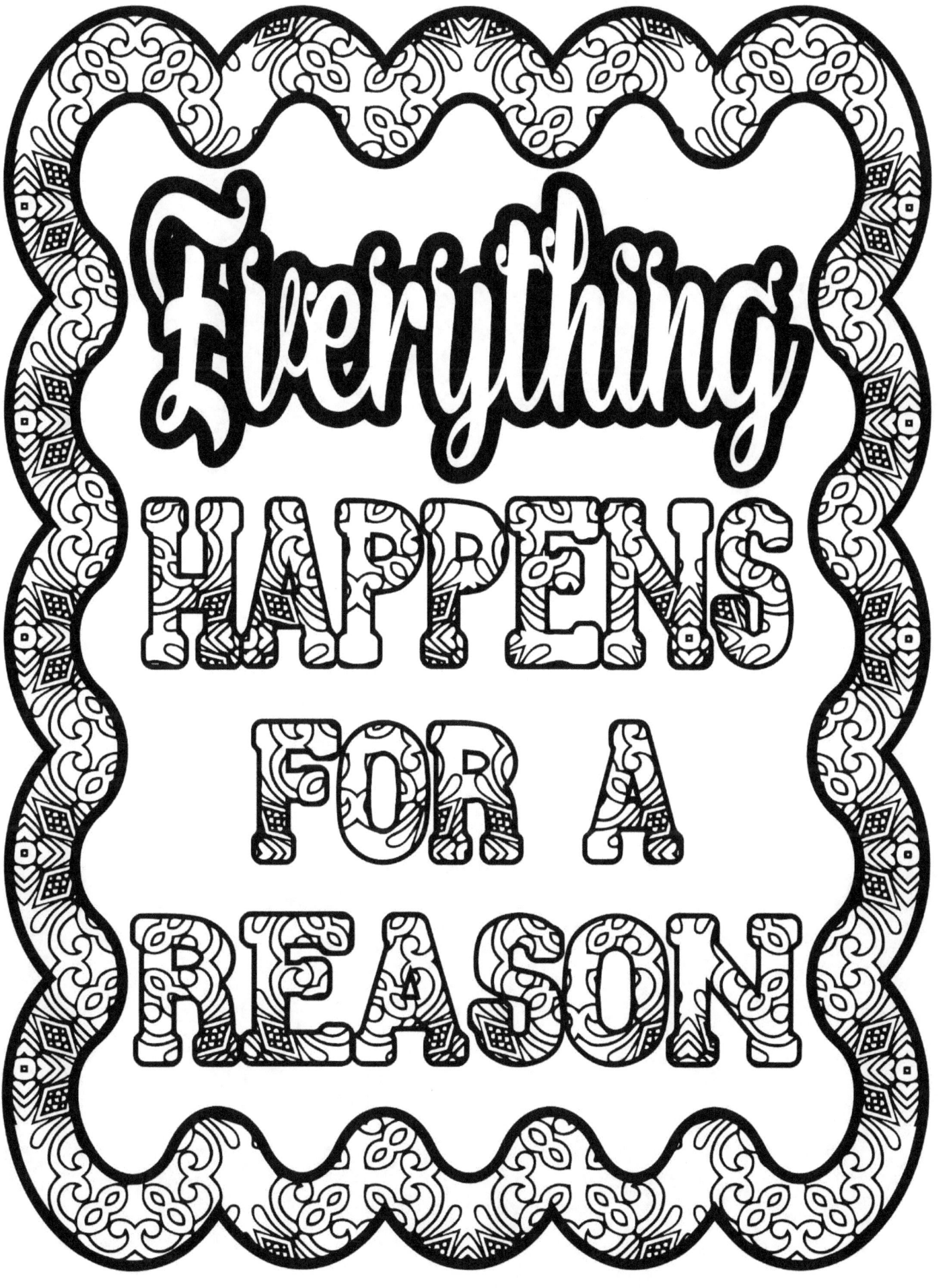

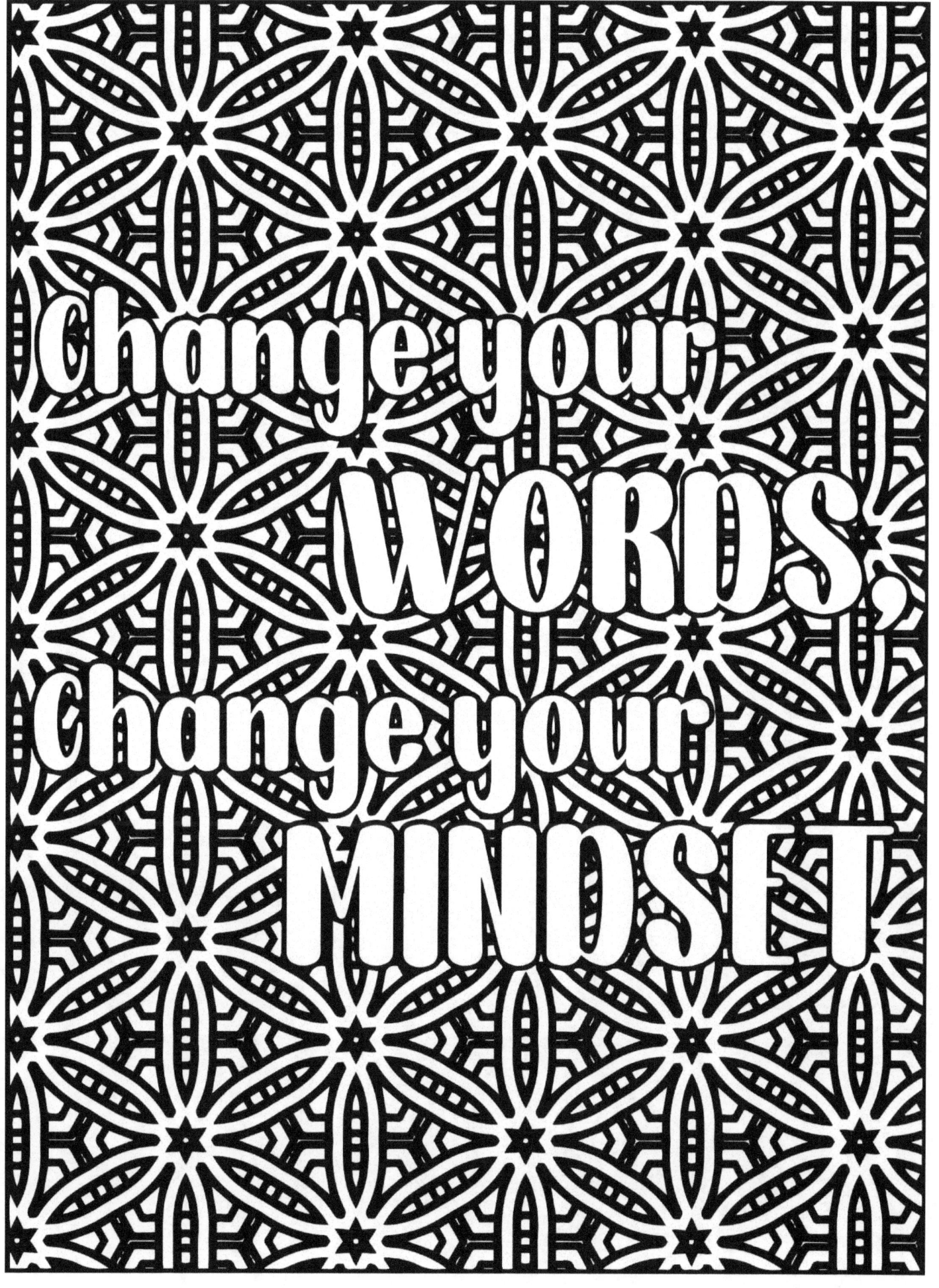

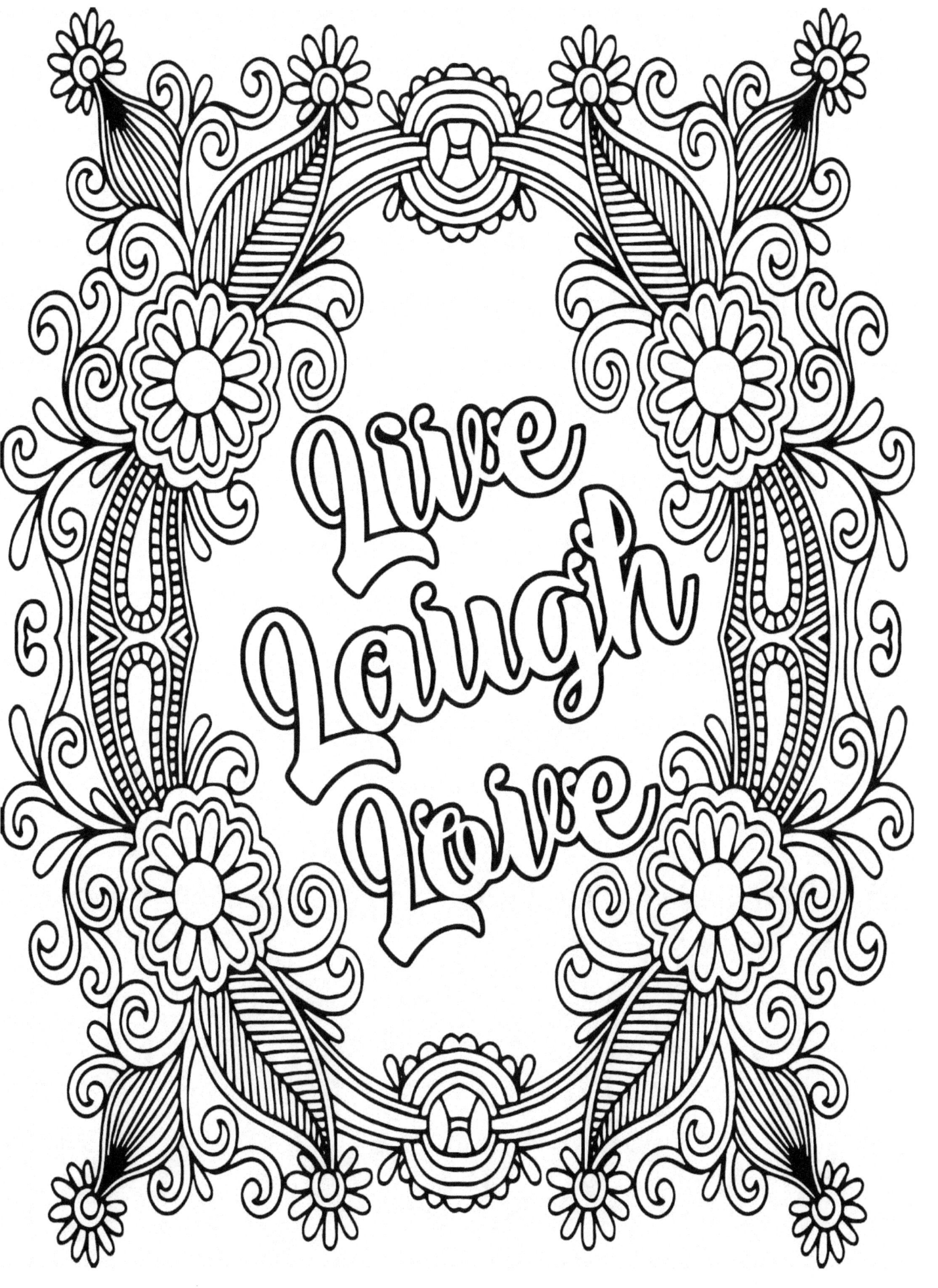

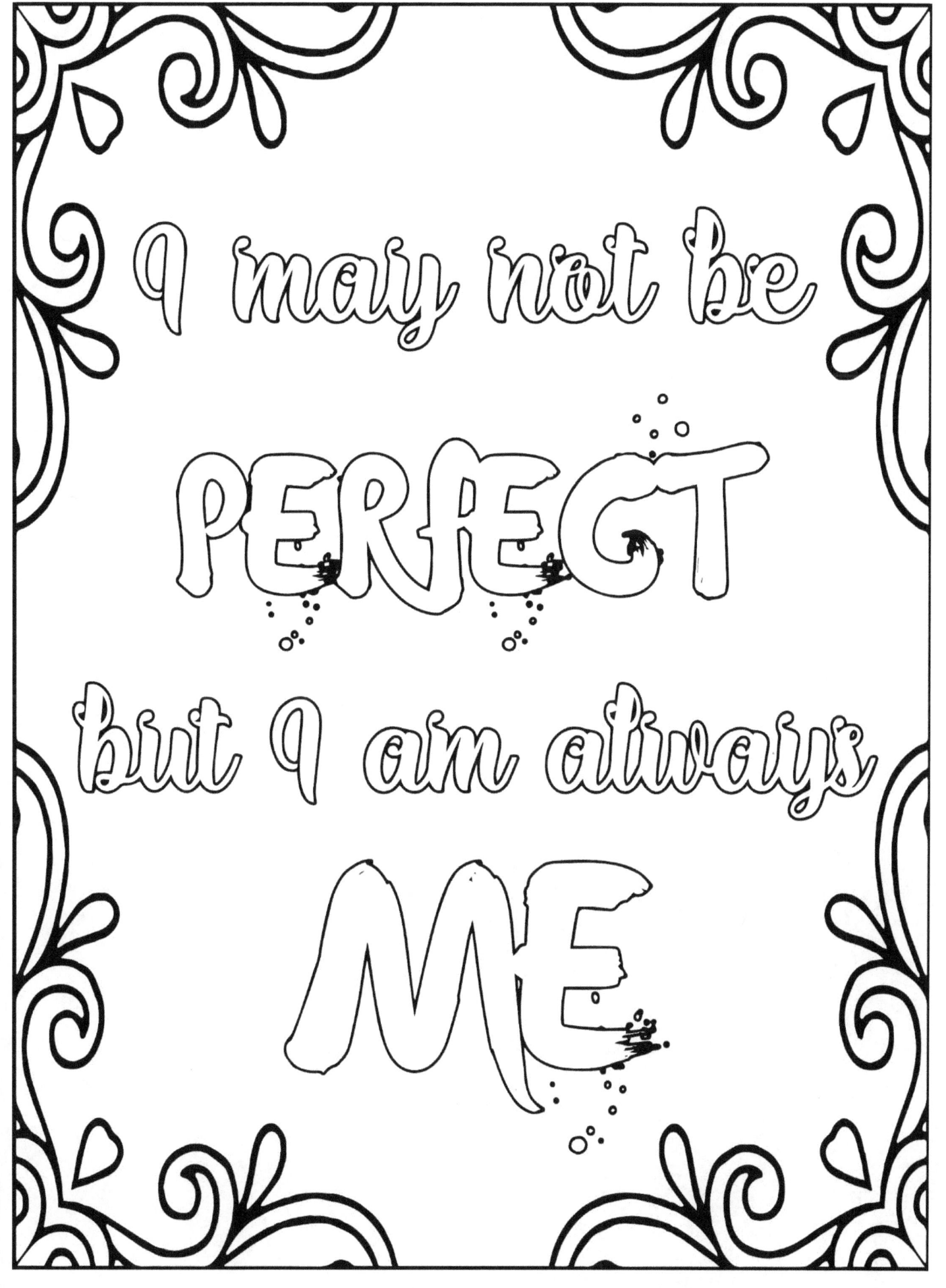

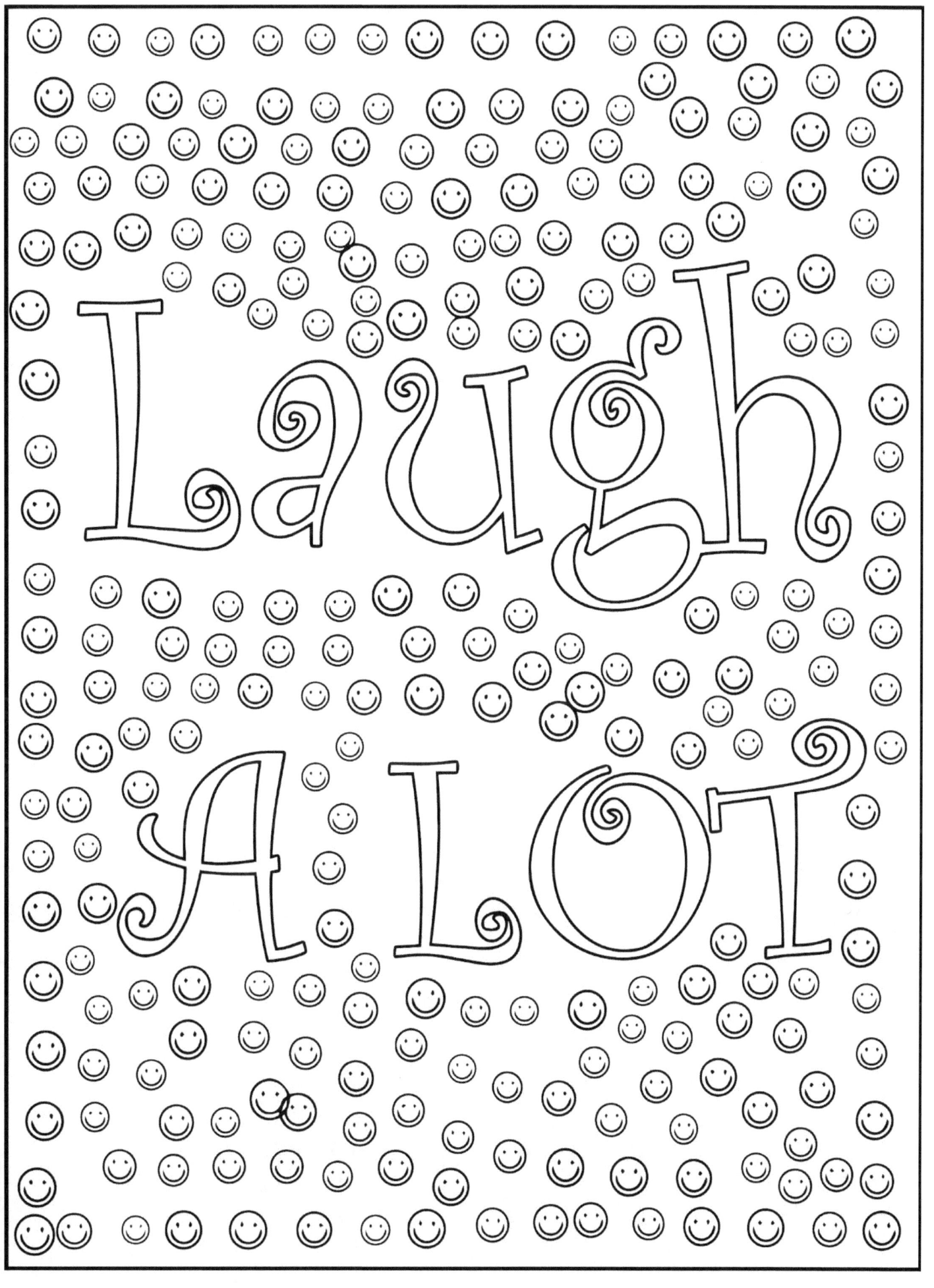

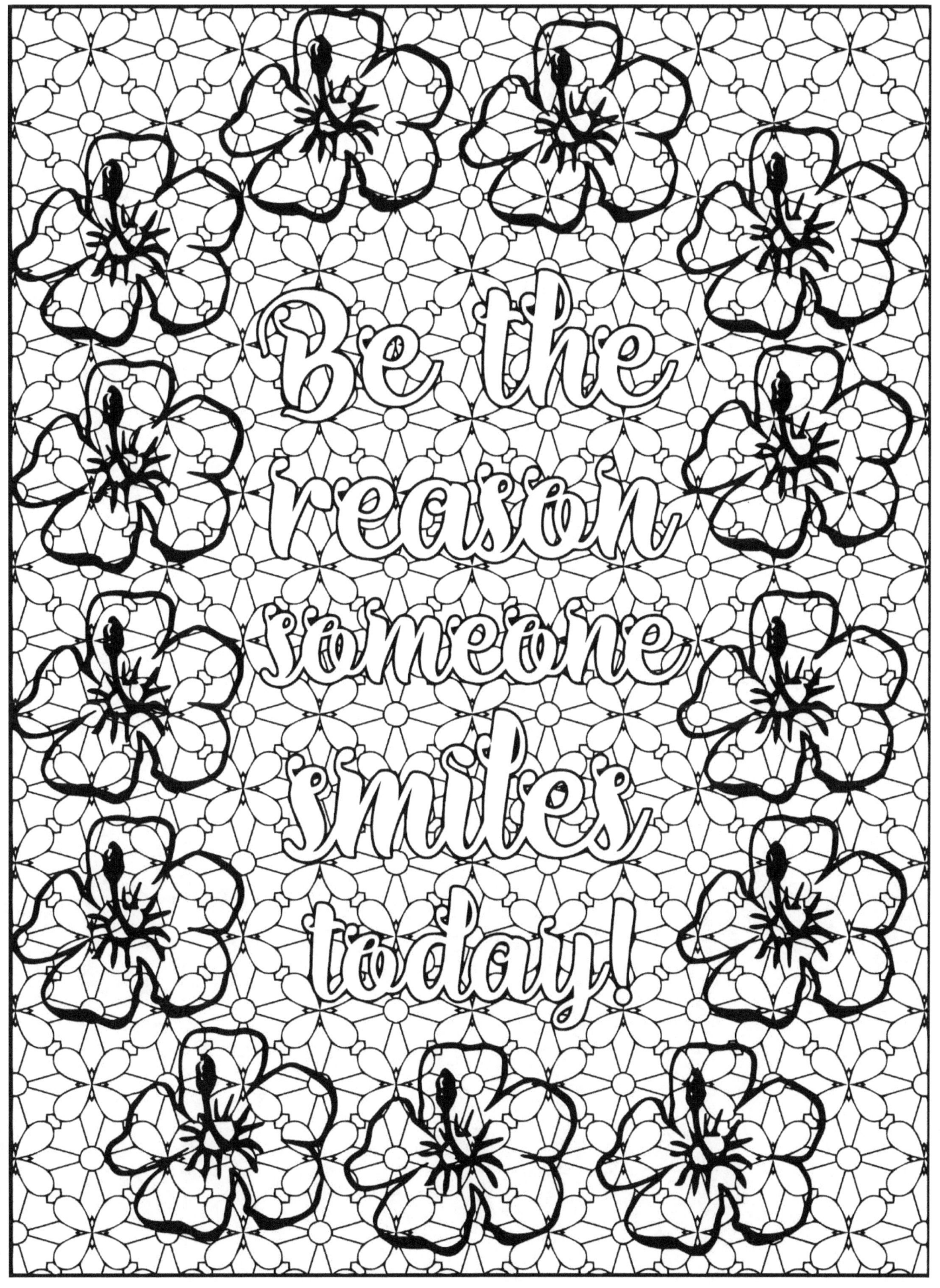

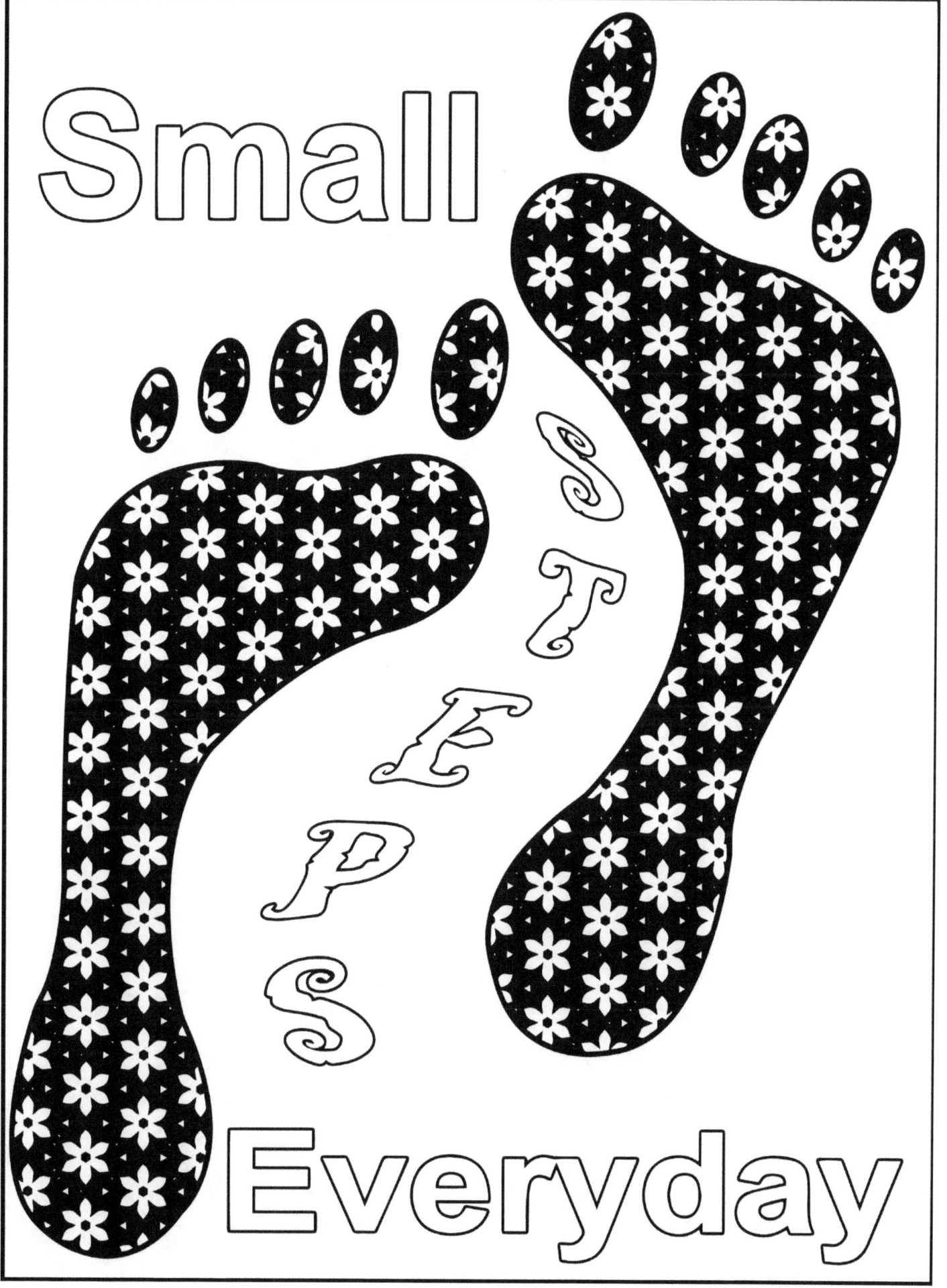

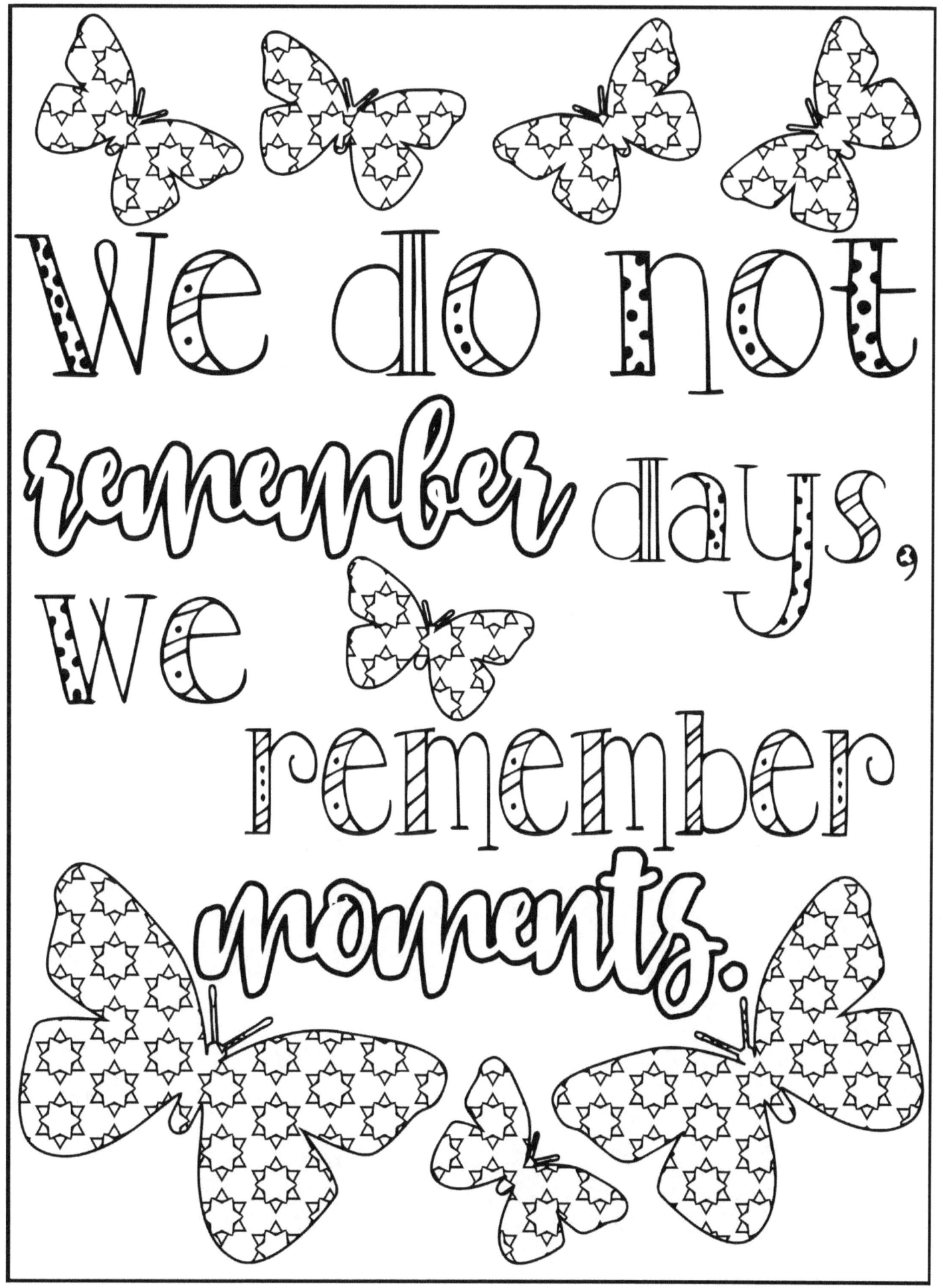

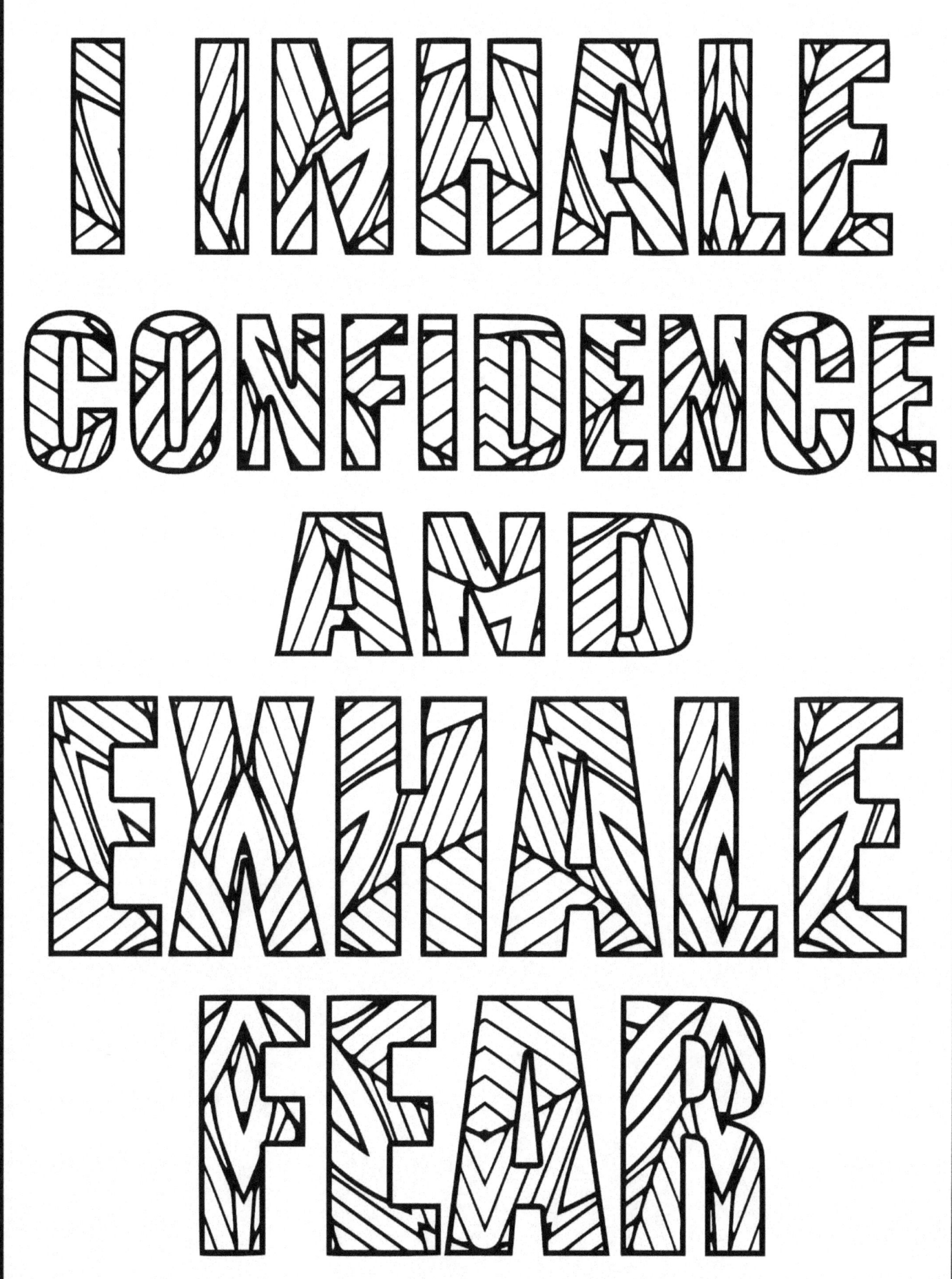

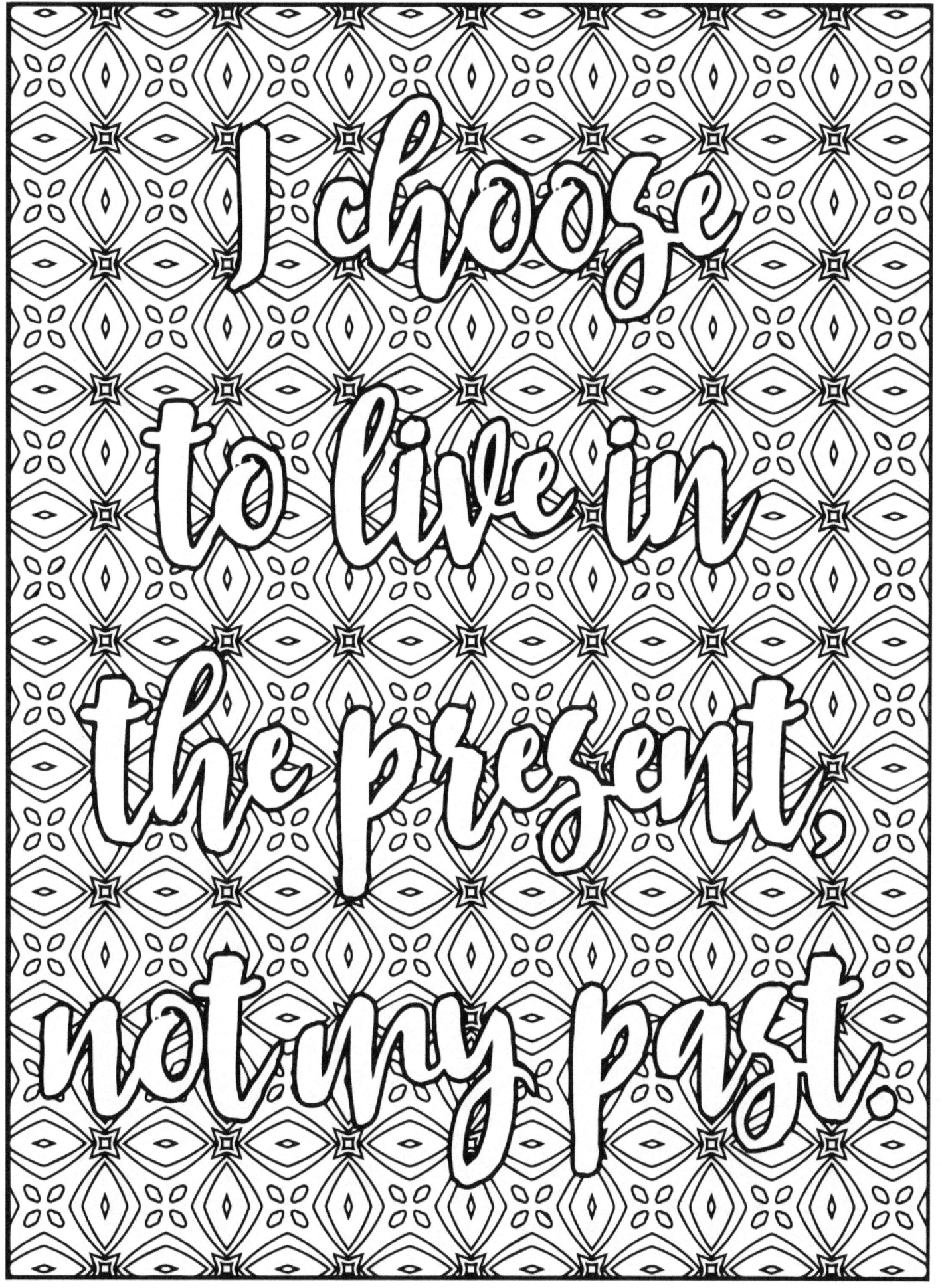

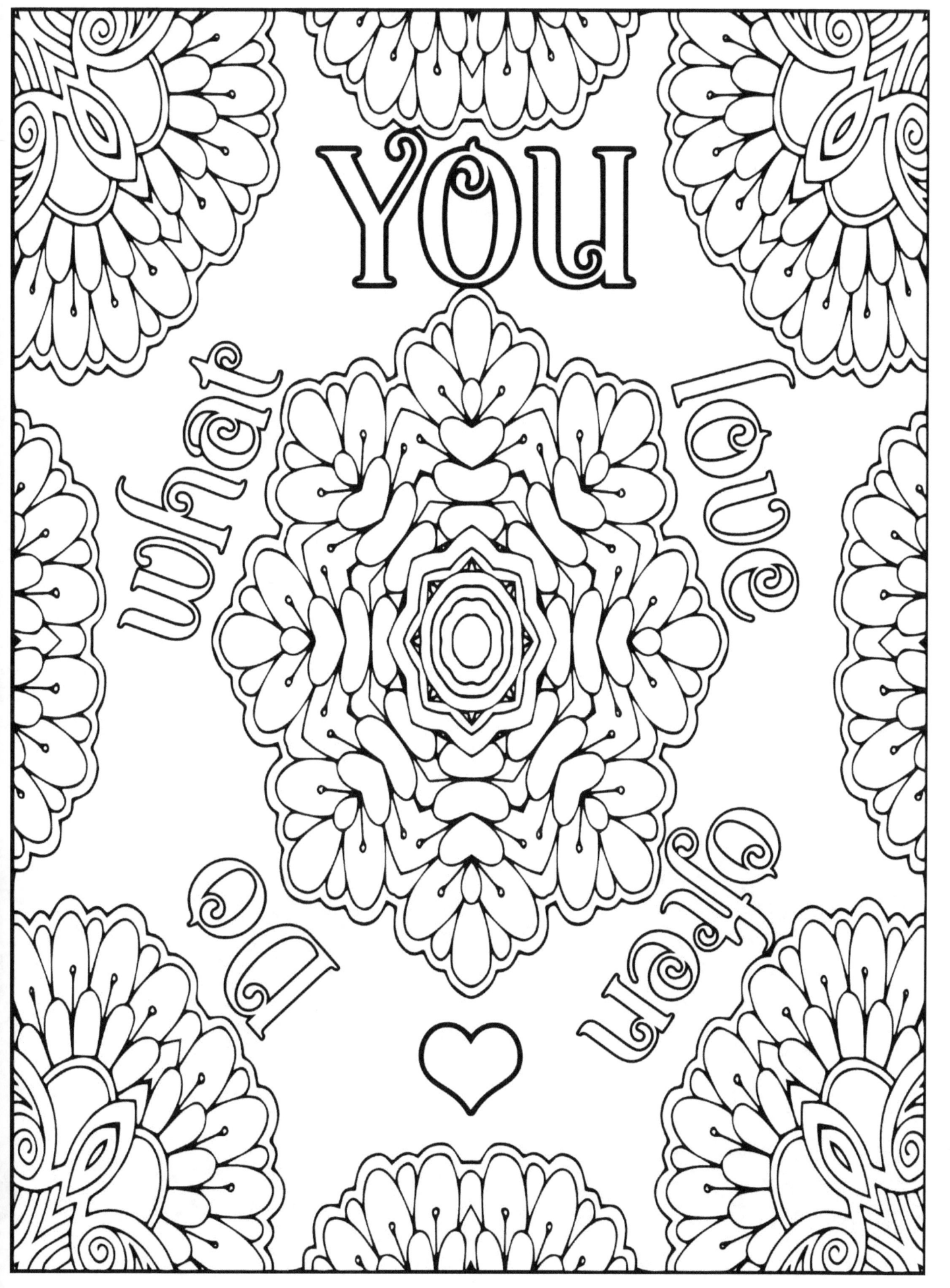

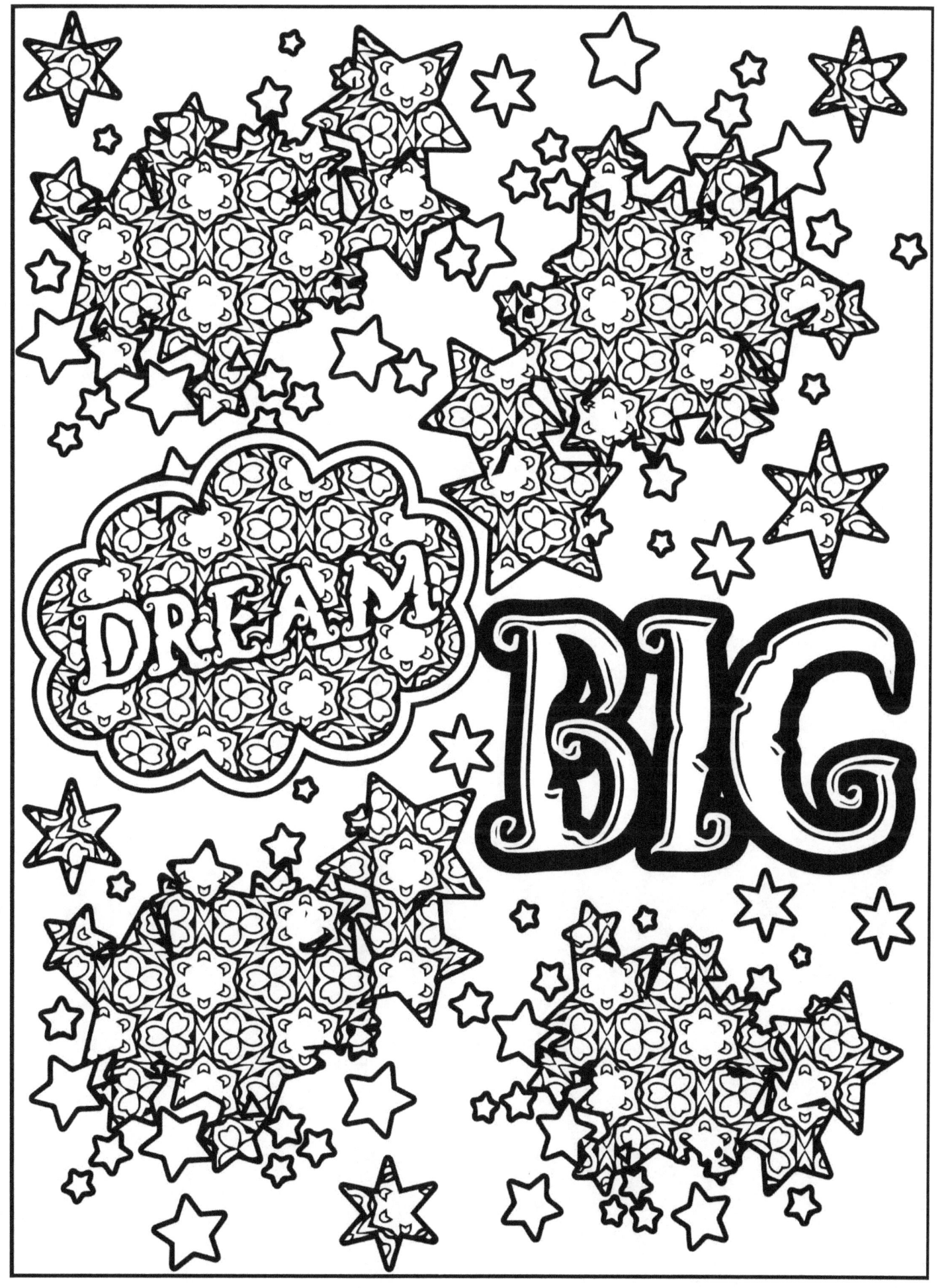

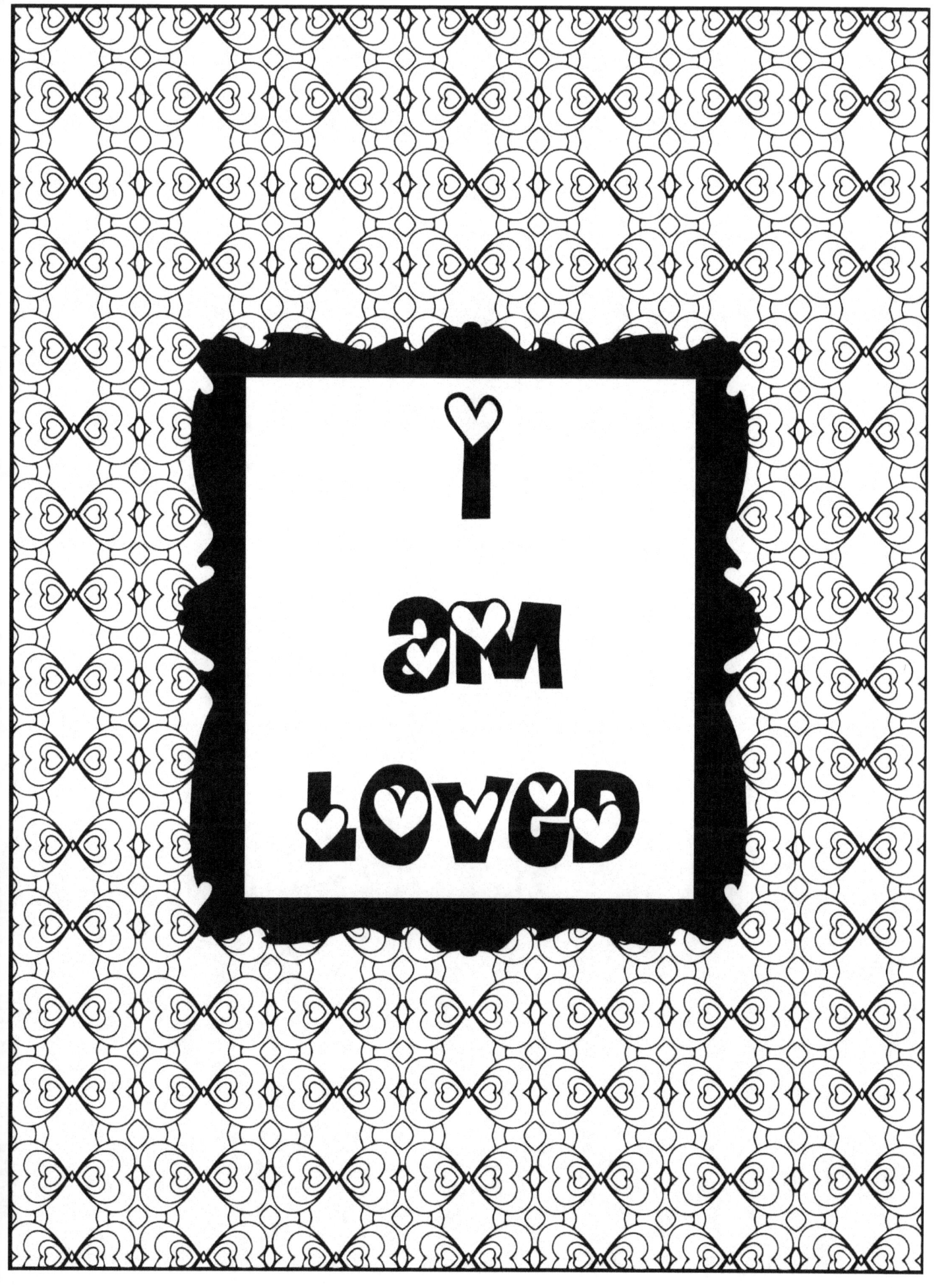

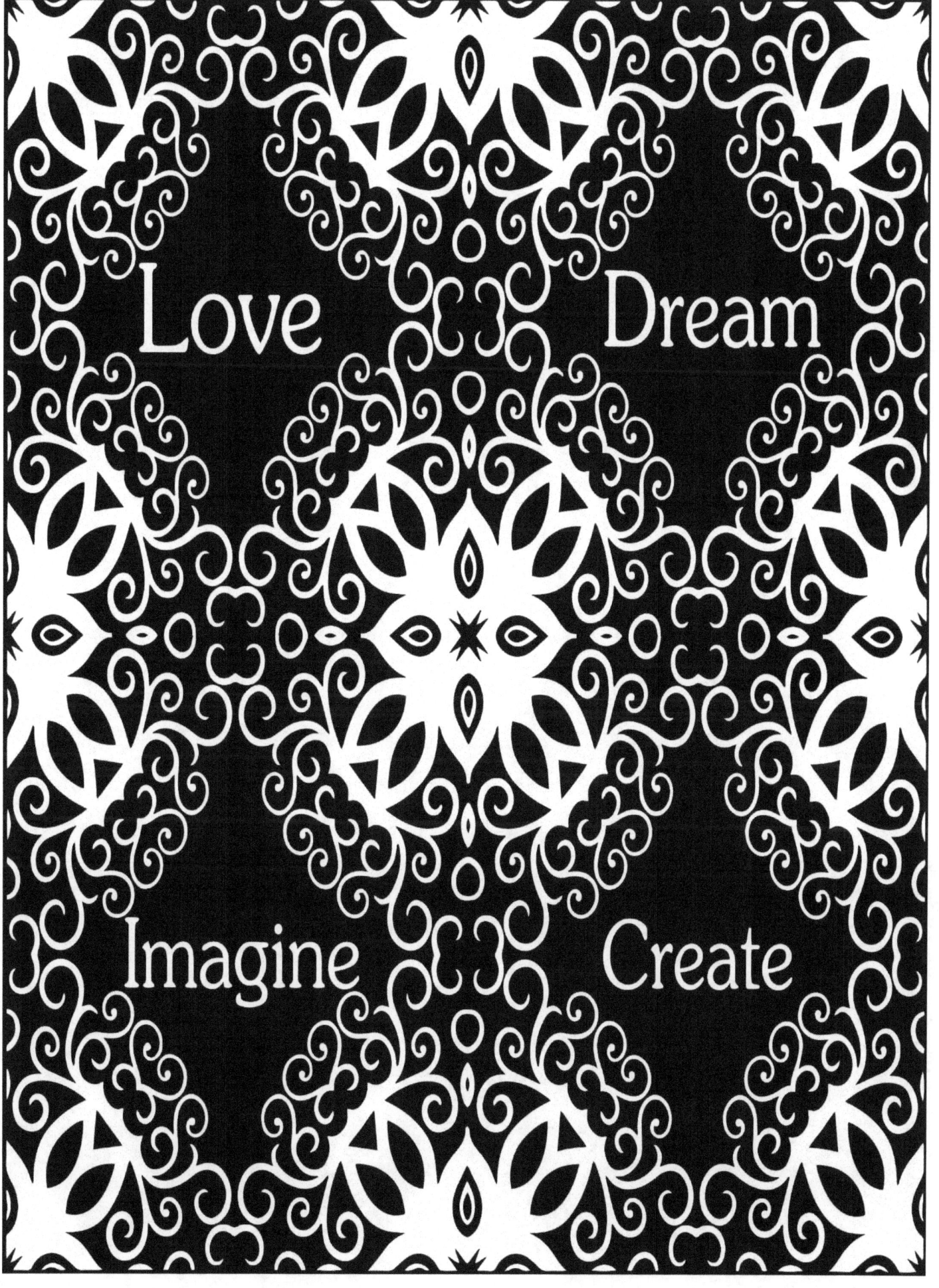

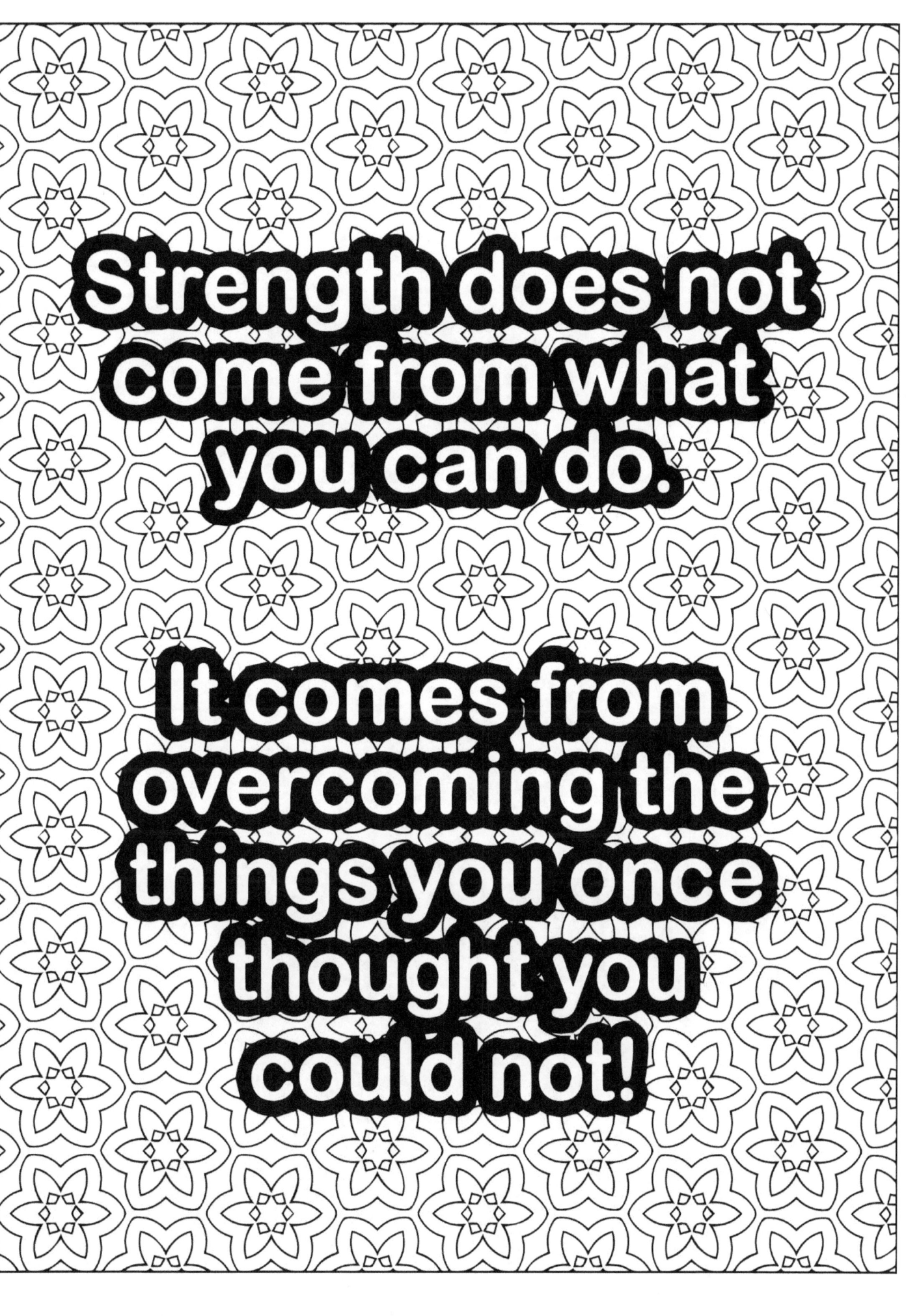

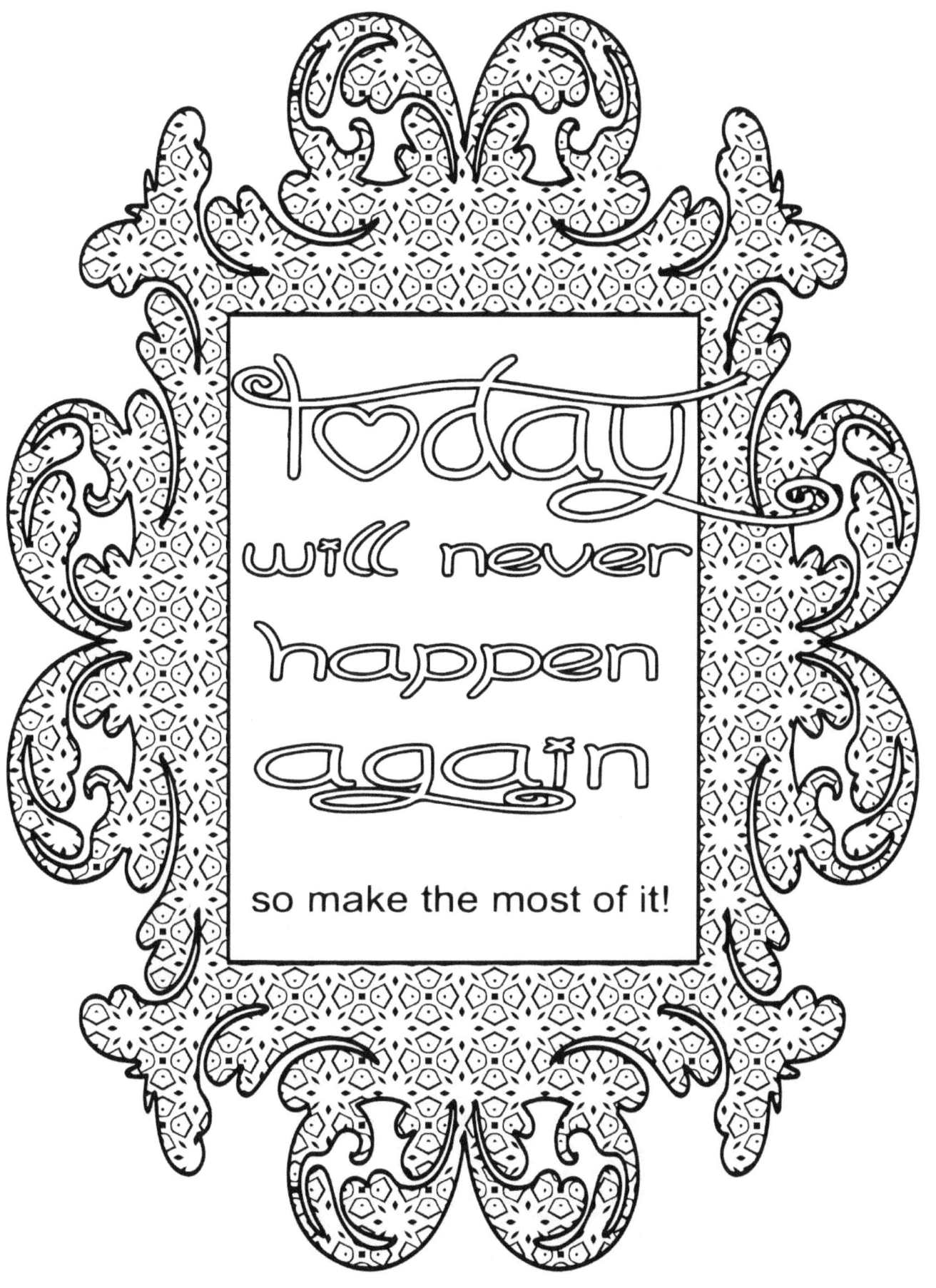

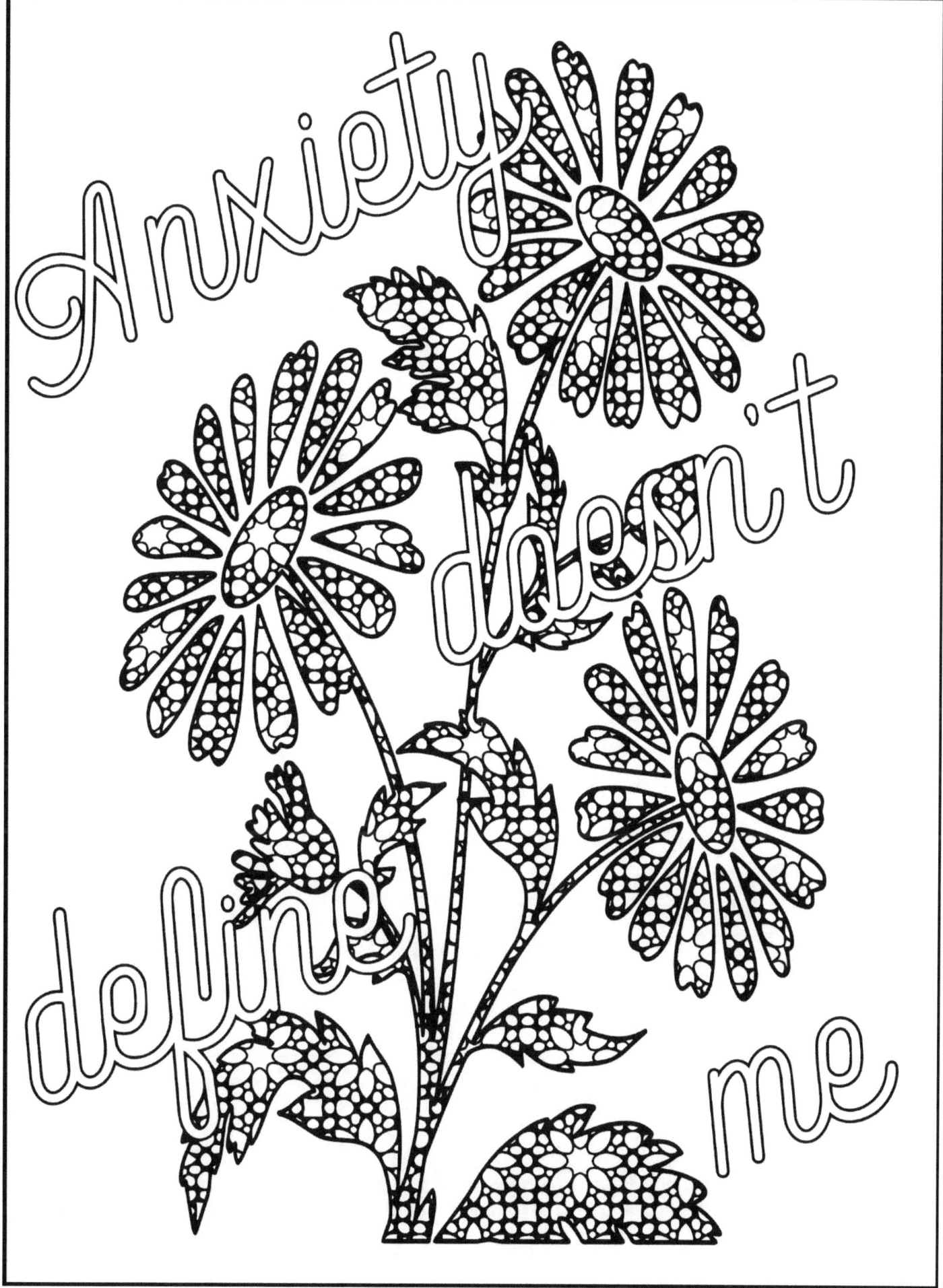

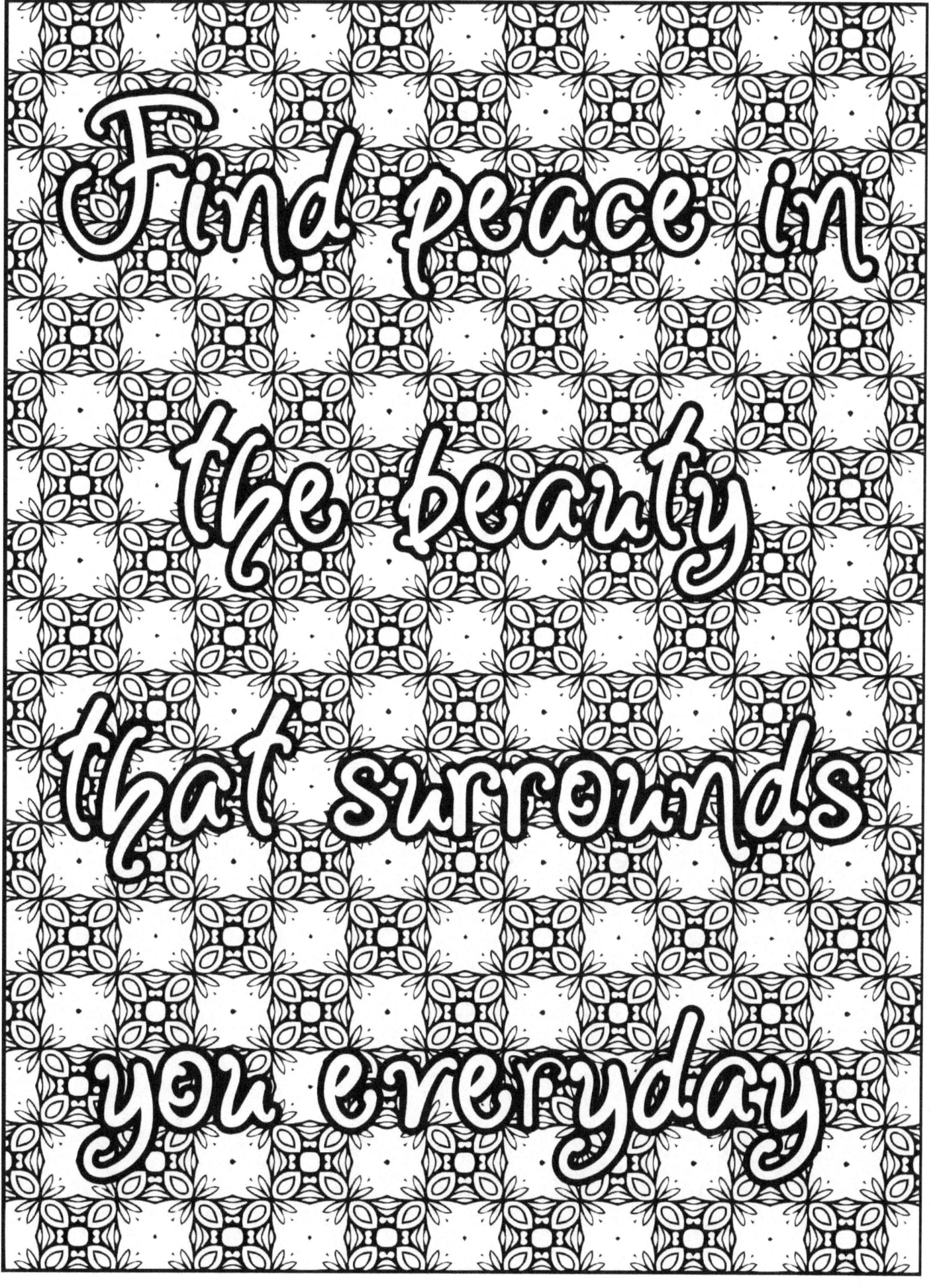

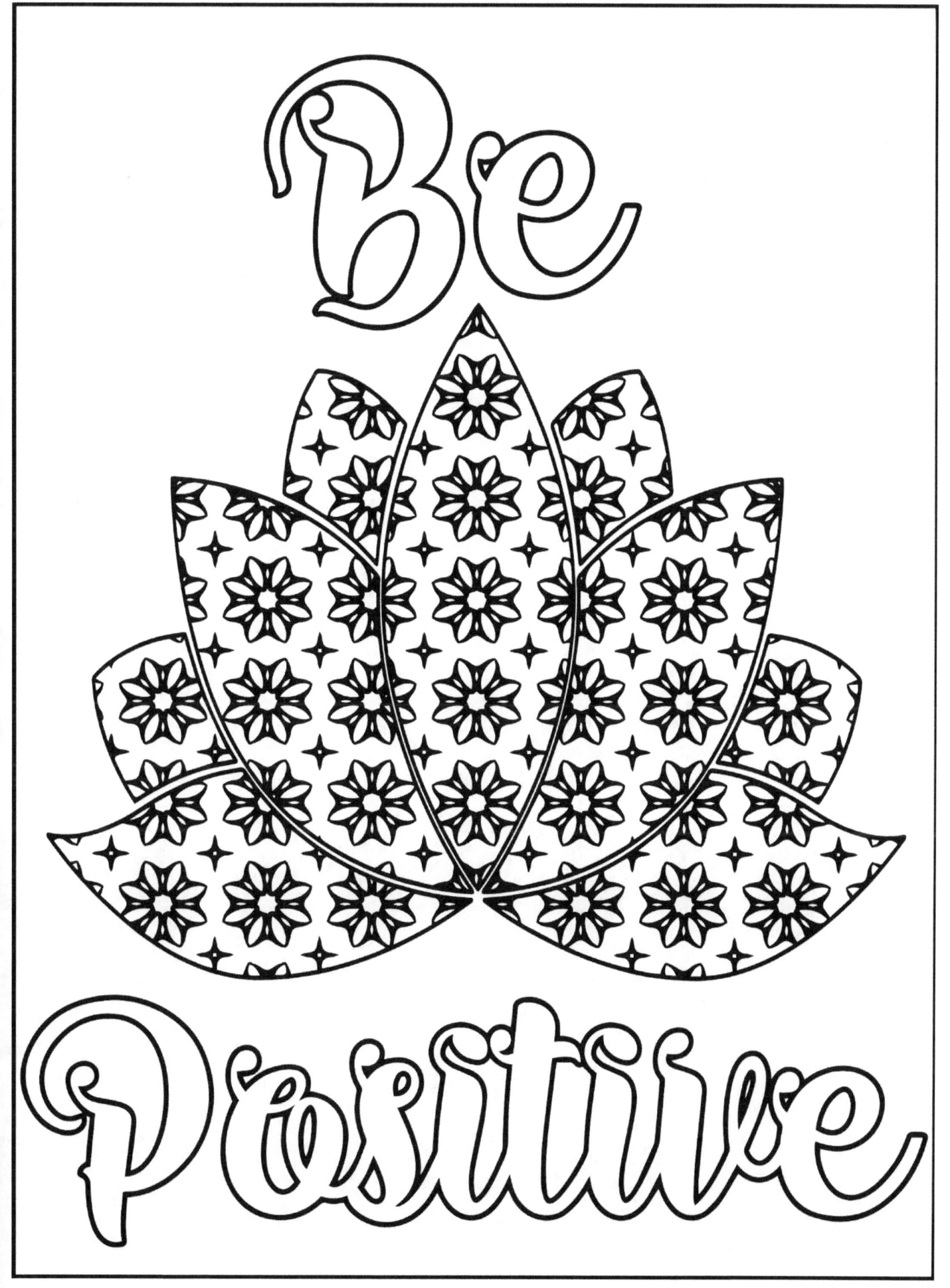

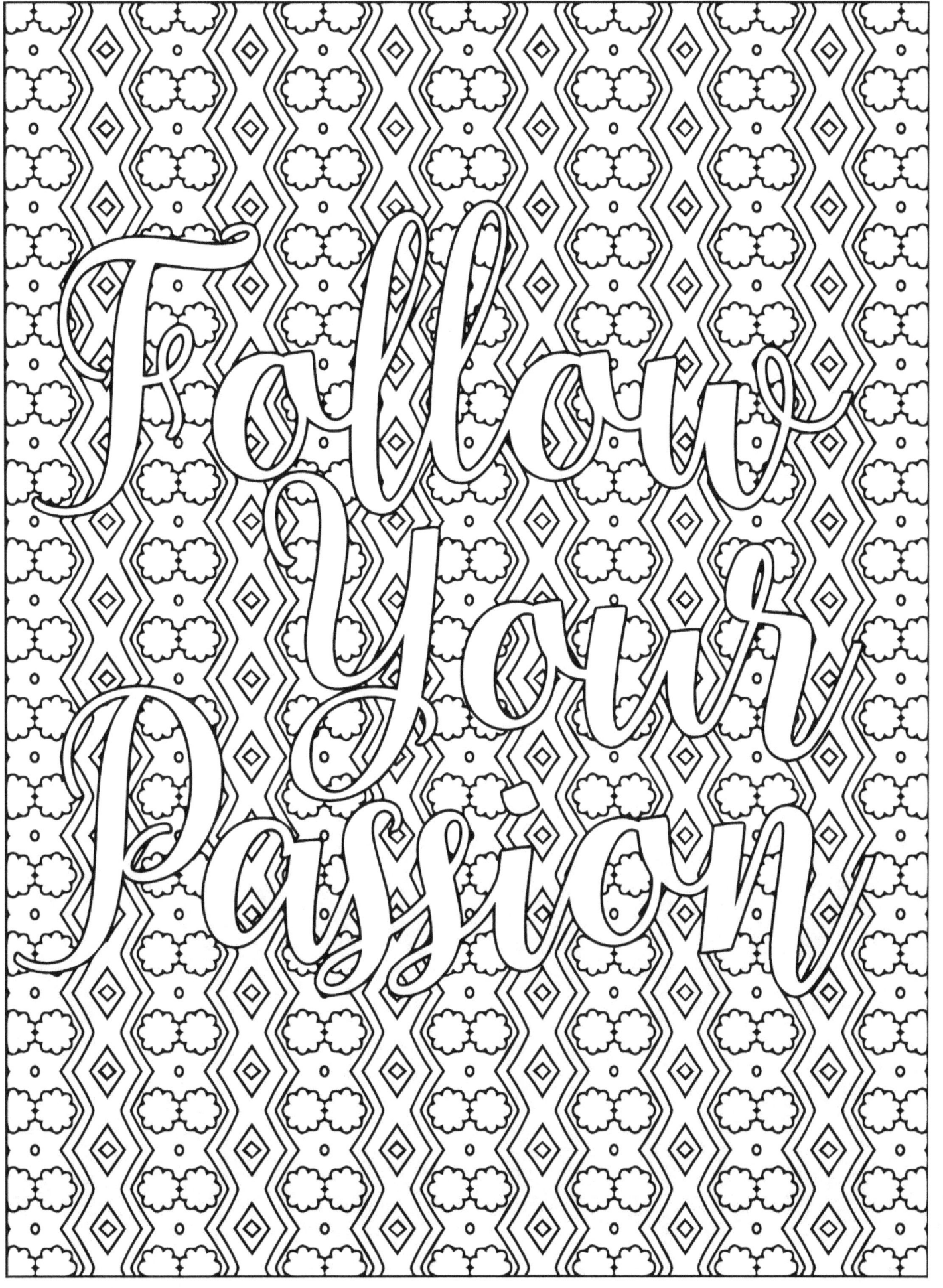

I only allow **HELPFUL** thoughts into my HEAD

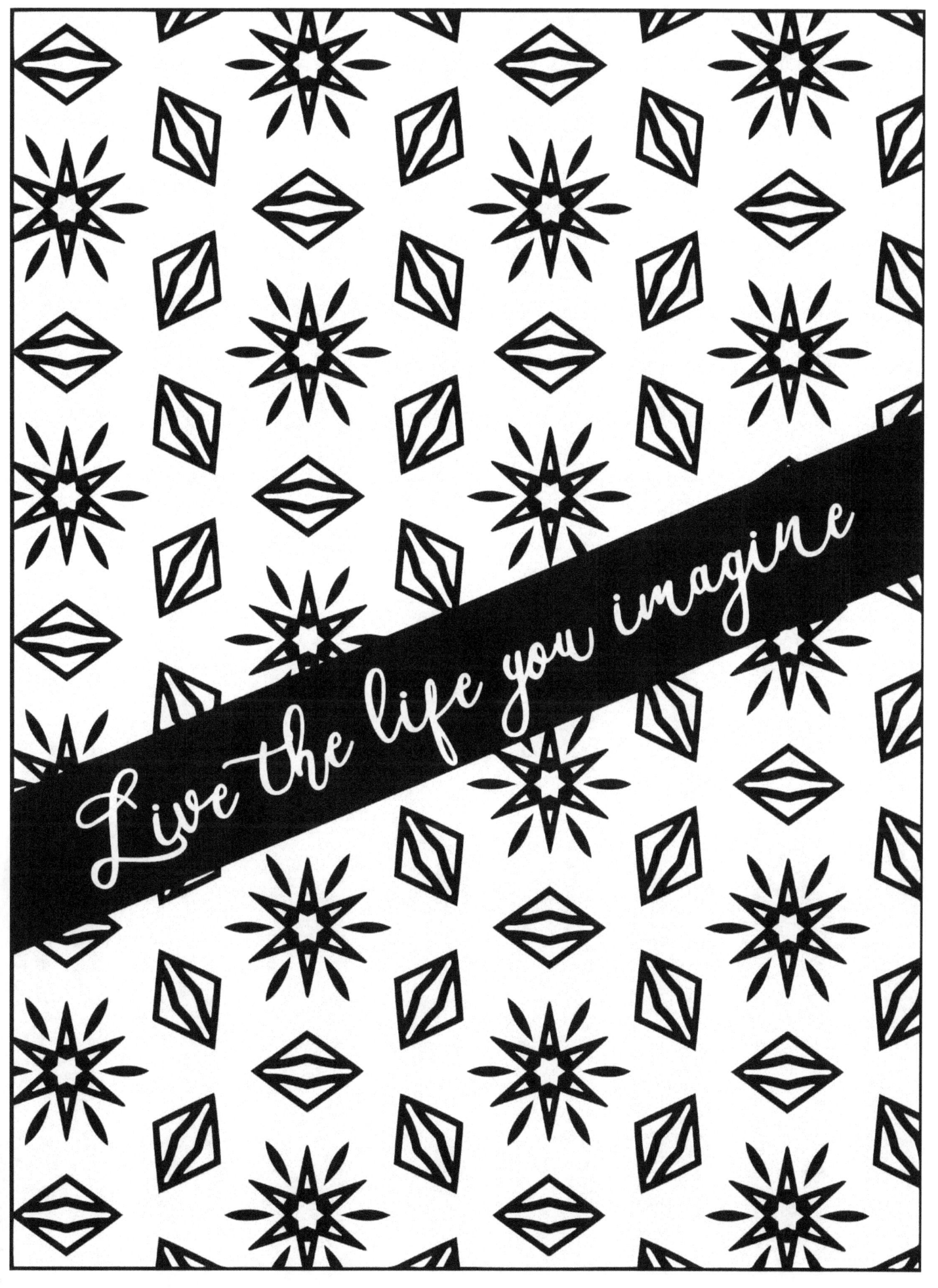

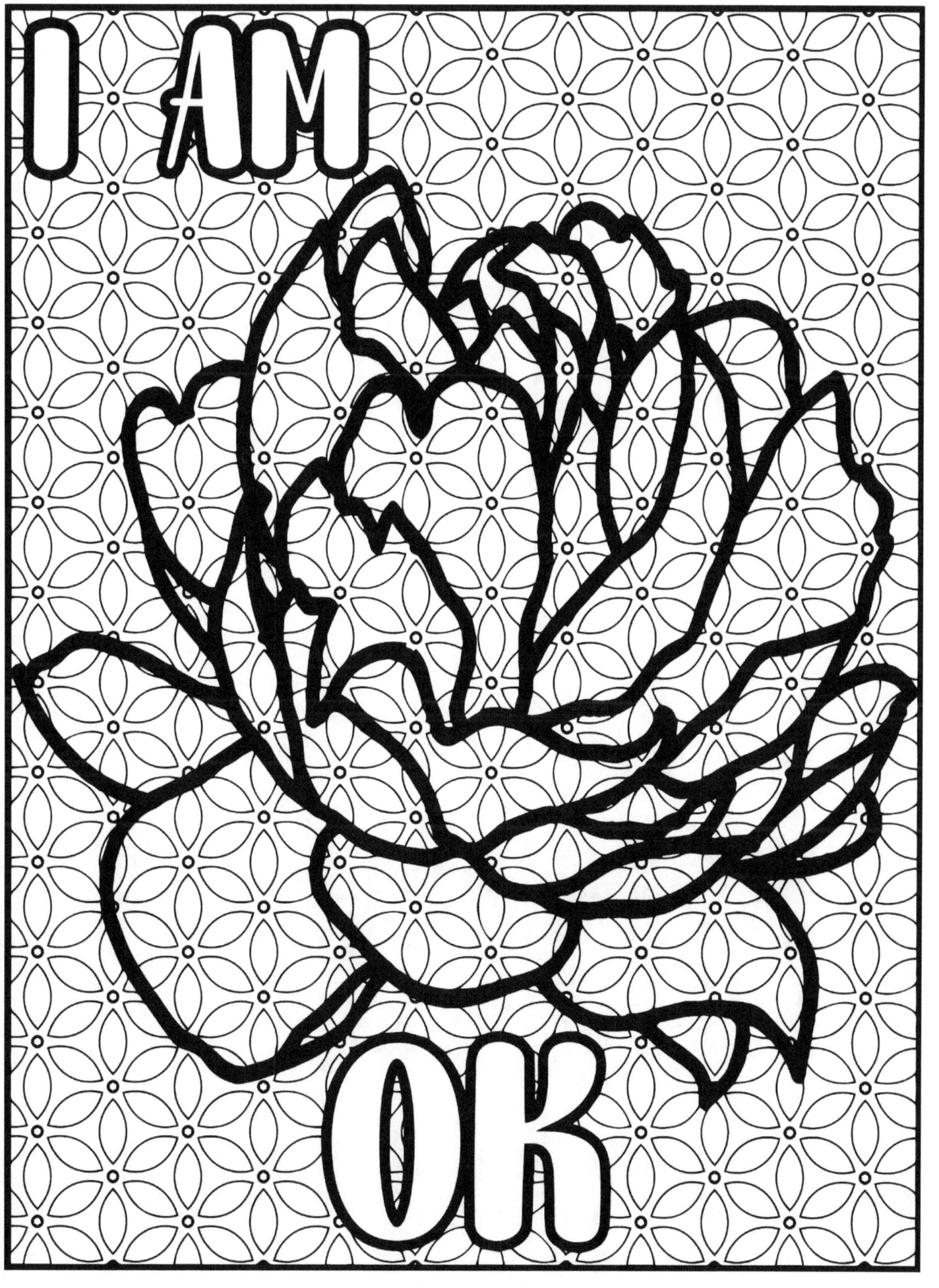

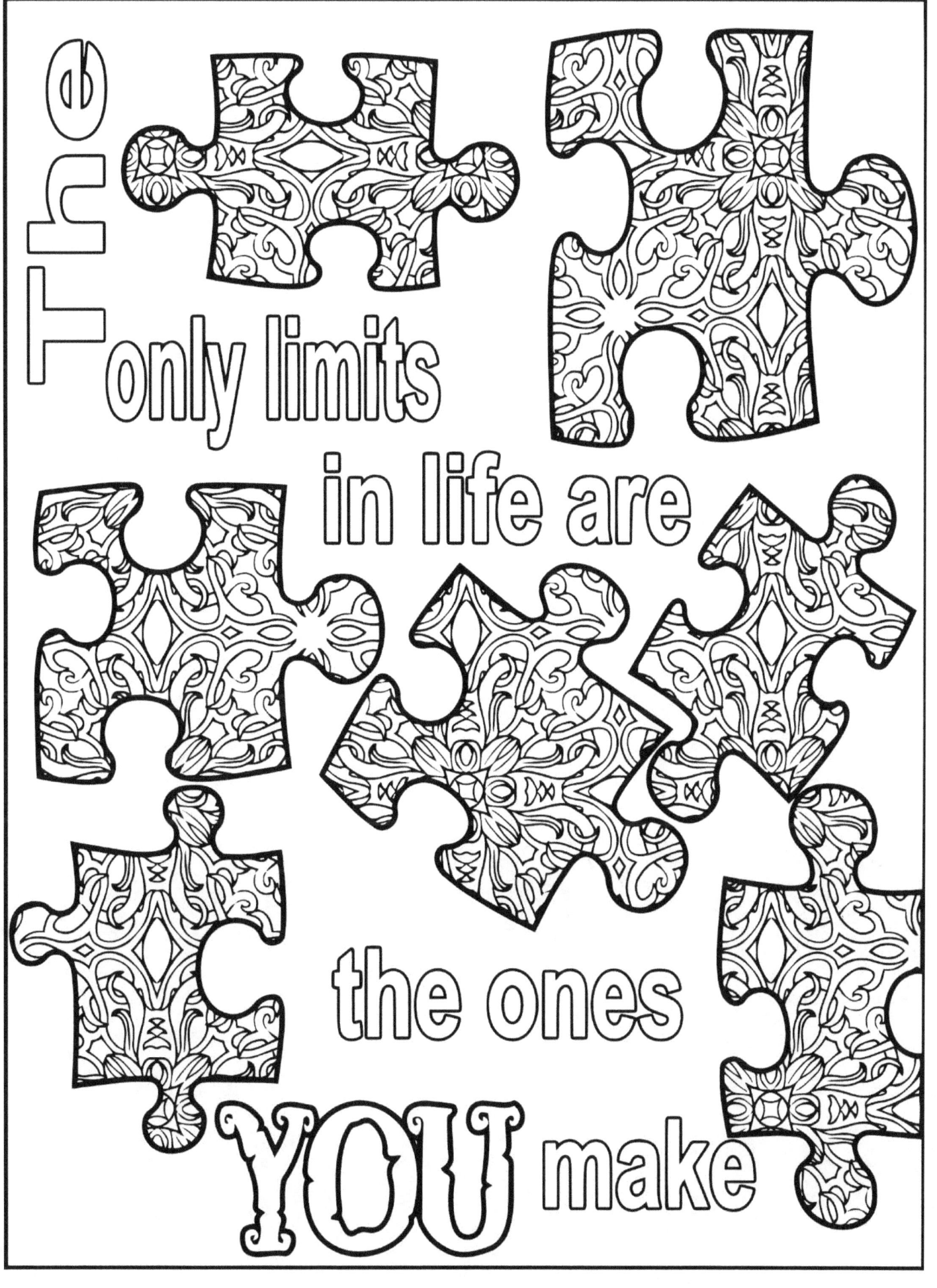

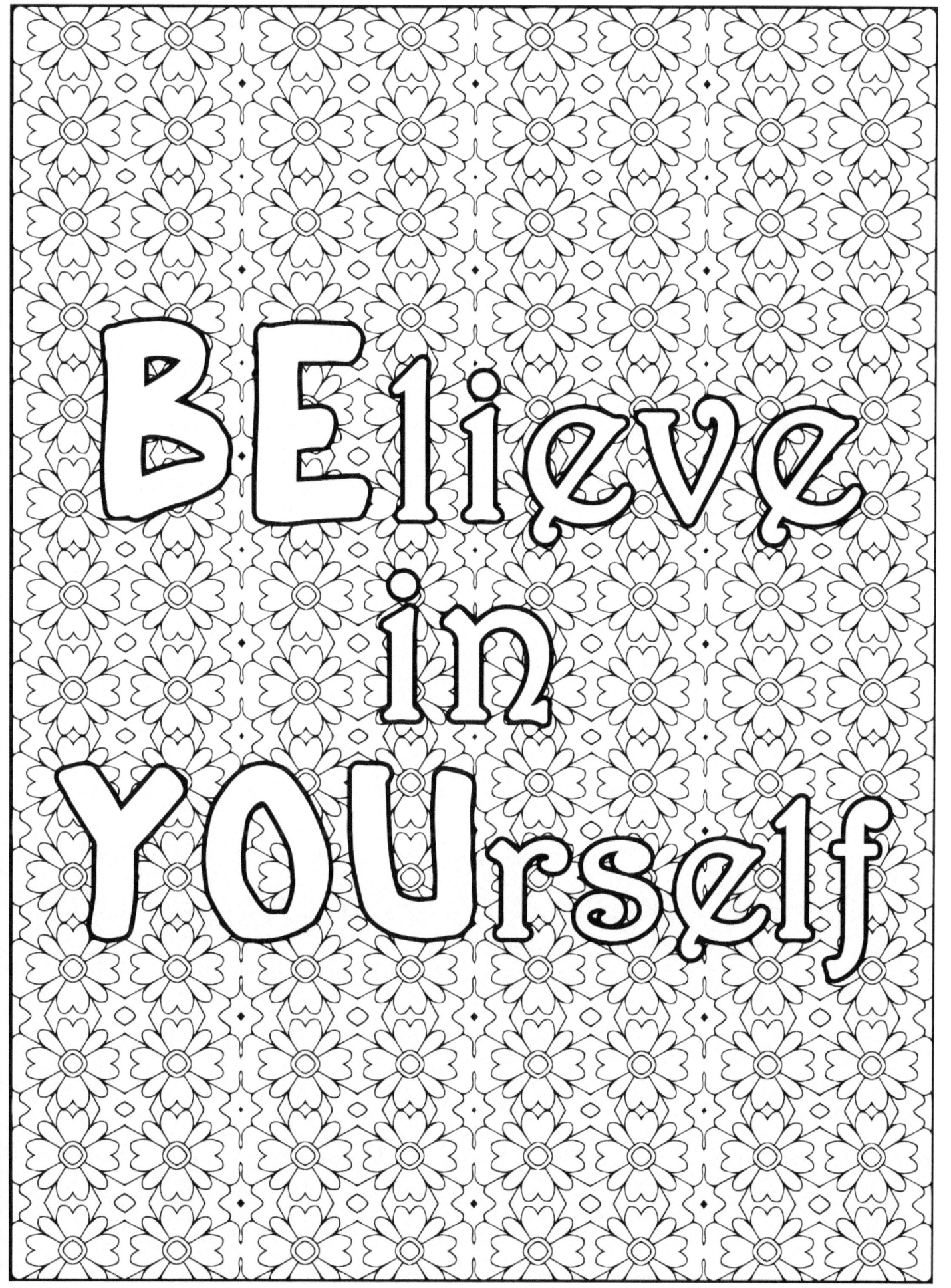

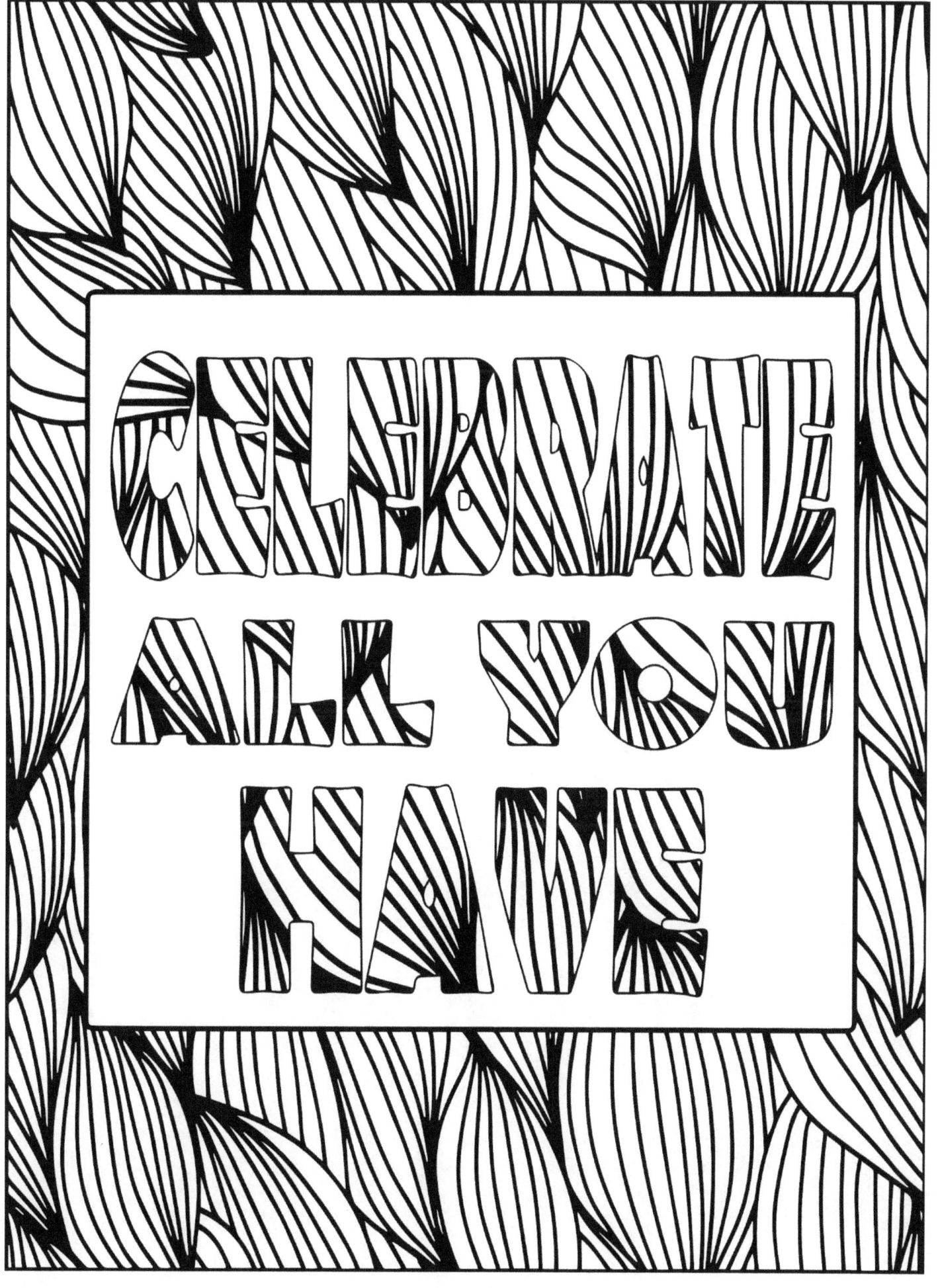

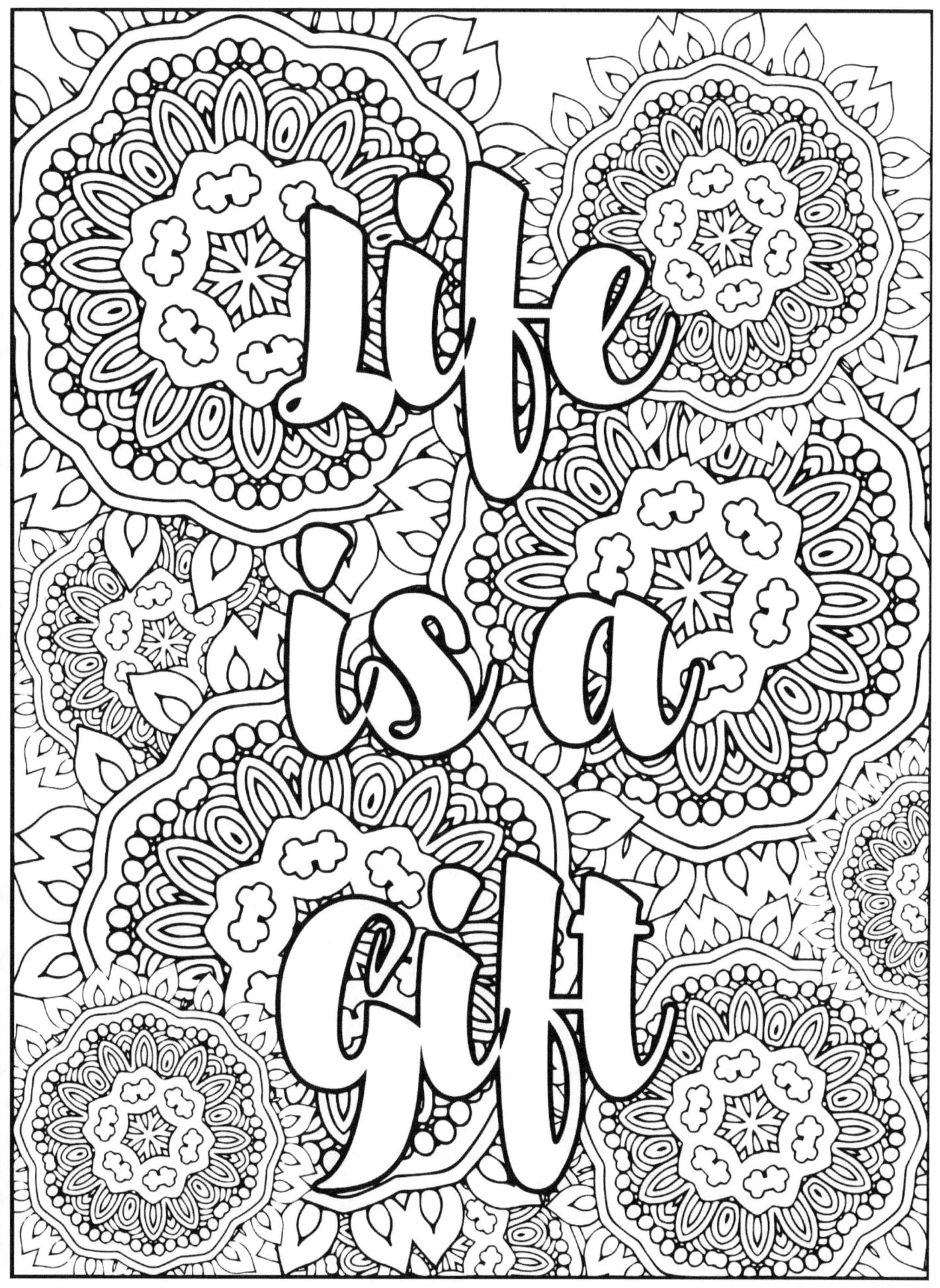

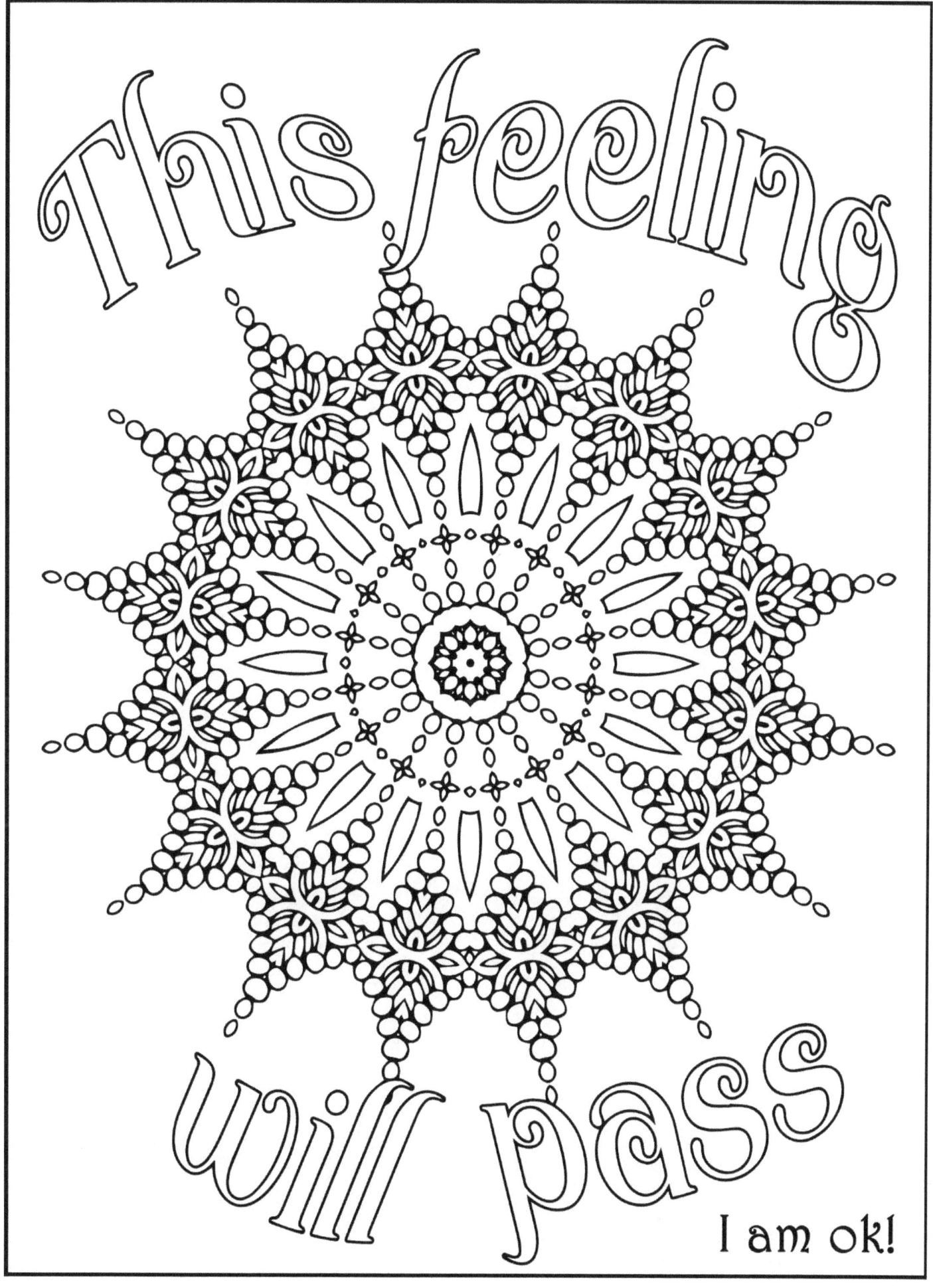

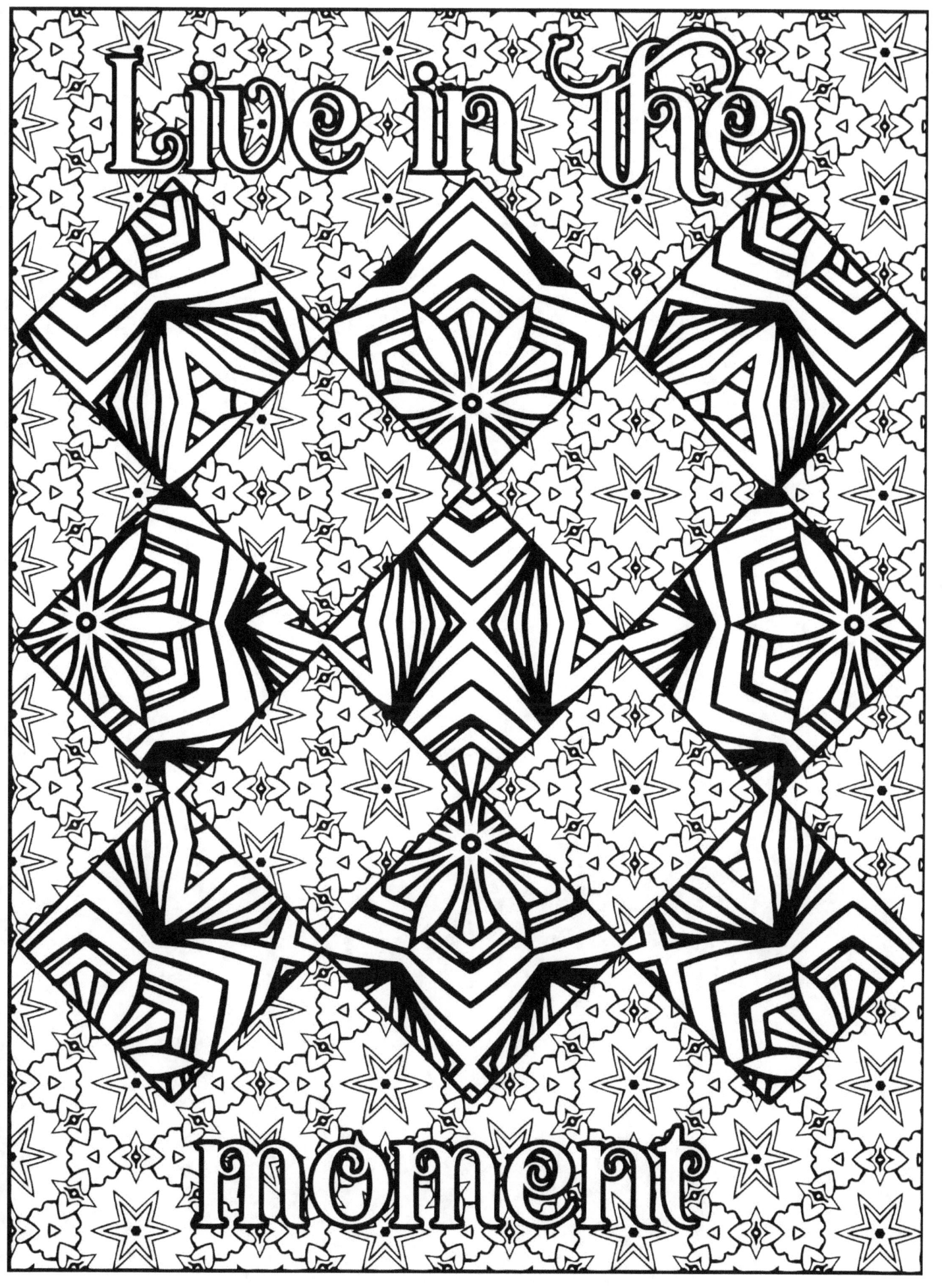

Bonus

Please enjoy these designs from the
Color Your Way To Happy
series of Adult Coloring Books

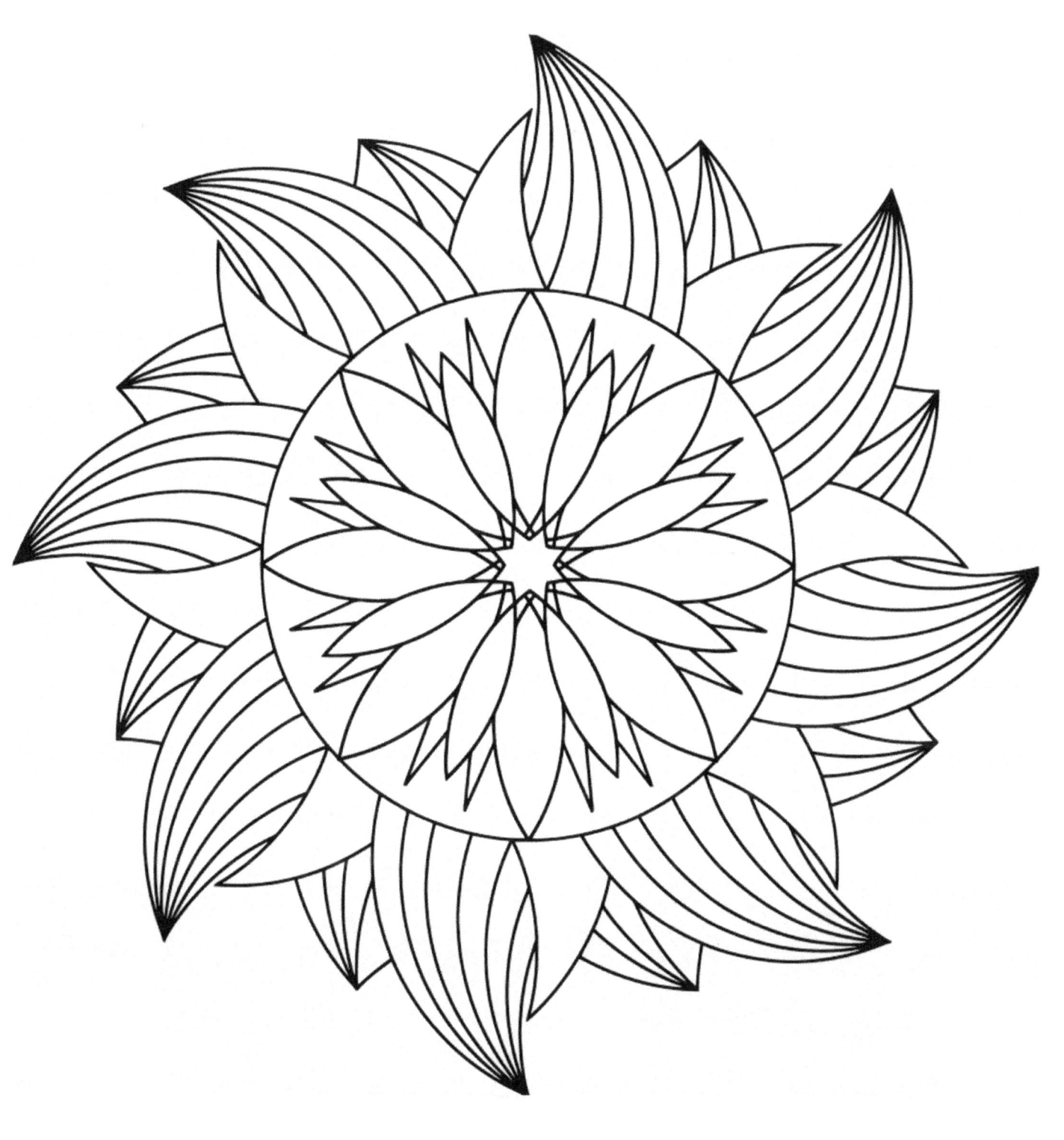

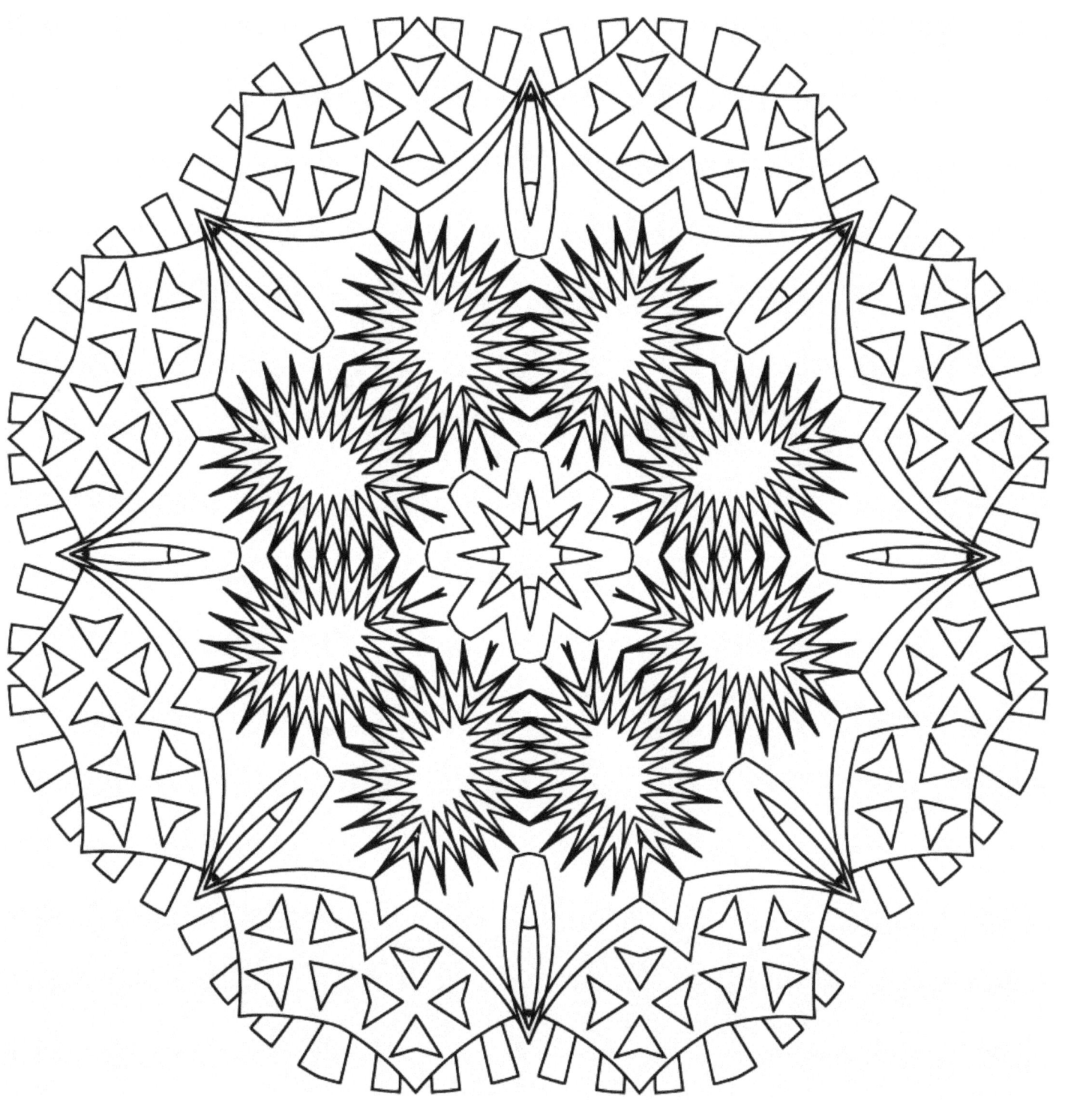

Sample from Mandalas for Mindfulness Volume 2 © Nerine Martin www.ColorYourWayToHappy.com

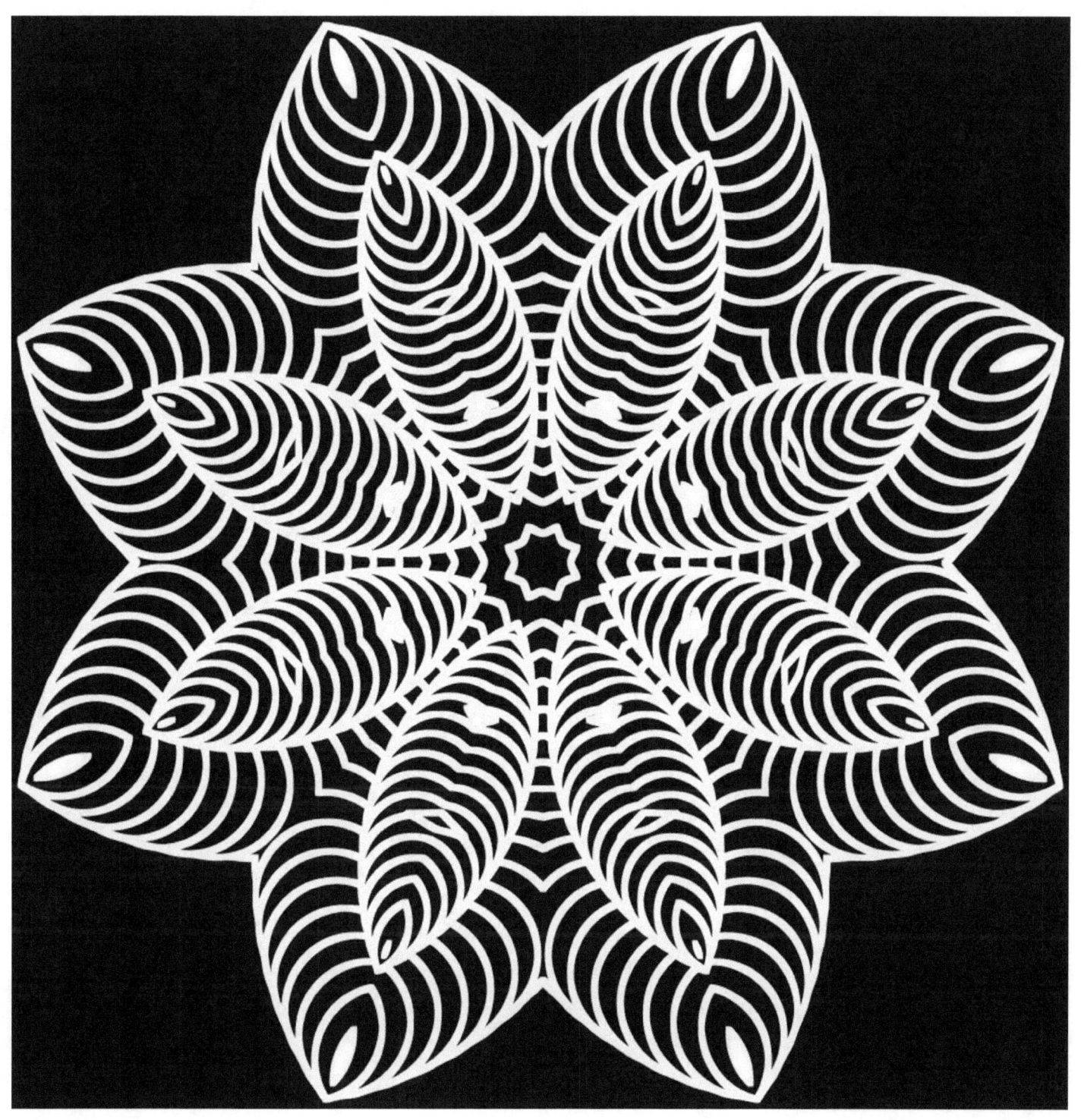

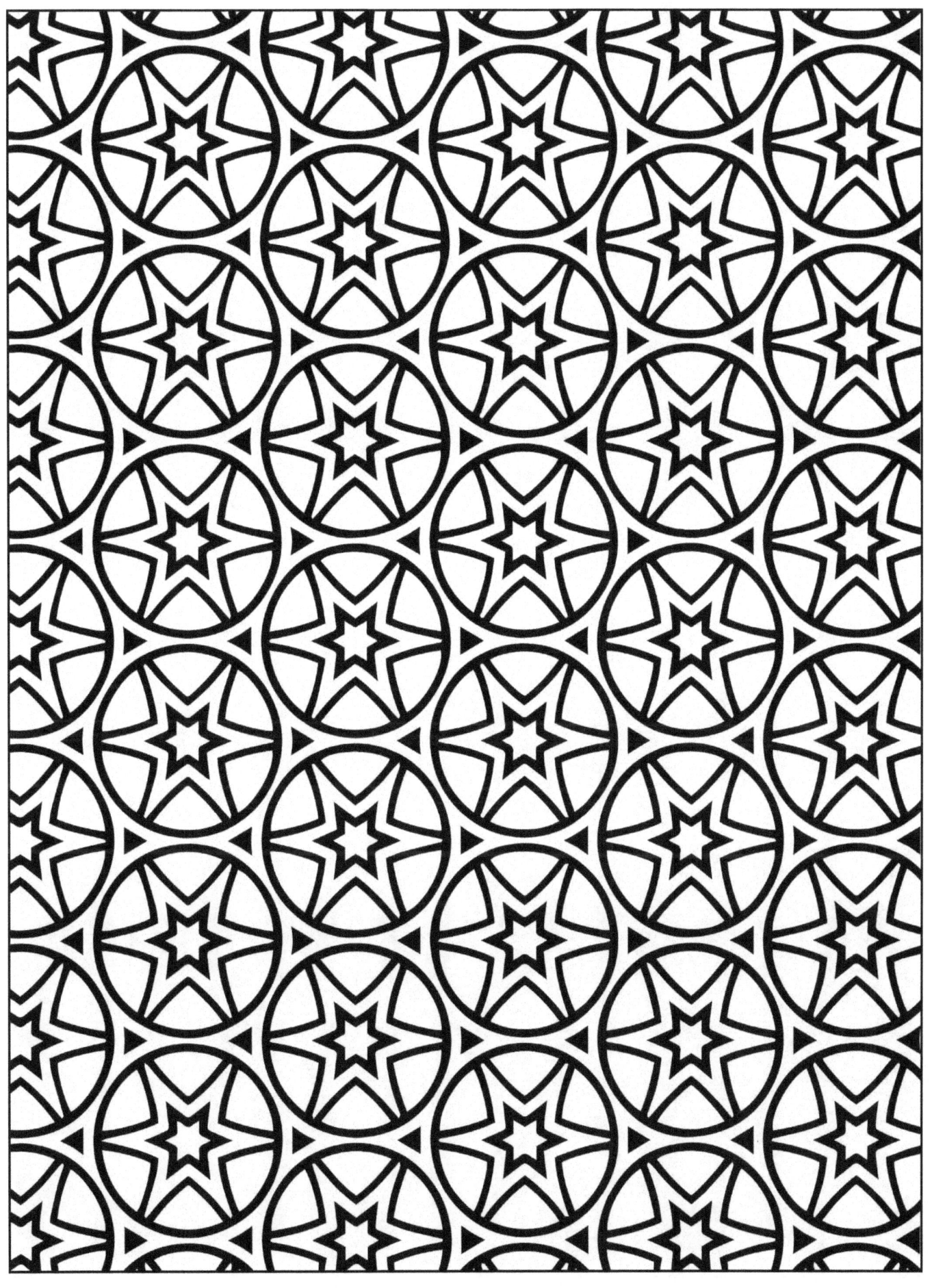

Stay In Touch & Explore More!

If you would like to be kept up-to-date with coloring tips, new book releases and news, and receive a FREE coloring book, please take the time to visit www.ColorYourWayToHappy.com/freebie and simply enter your details.

Remember to Like, Share & Comment on my Facebook page and feel free to let your friends and family know about my page too. I would love it if you shared your finished colored pages with me and join in the conversations with other coloring enthusiasts.

Just go to: **www.facebook.com/ColorYourWayToHappy**

******

I truly appreciate you purchasing my coloring books, so could I please ask a small favor of you?

Would you take just a moment to leave an honest review of my coloring book? It doesn't have to be long, just a sentence or two that tells people what you liked about the book.

Your words and 5 stars will go a long way to letting other readers know they'll like this coloring book too!

Add your review on Amazon at **www.ColorYourWayToHappy.com/Anxiety**

Thanks again and remember to have fun and 'Color Your Way To Happy'!

Nerine ☺

P.S. Did you know you can also purchase a PDF instant downloadable version of this coloring book to print at home? This is a great way to print your favorite pages as many times as you like, to color over and over, or to print onto cardstock. You can also purchase a downloadable version of all my coloring books at a discounted price at www.ColorYourWayToHappy.com.

About The Artist

Nerine Martin was born in Perth, Australia and loves all things crafty and colorful. From trying her hand at many crafts including her all-time favorites of scrapbooking and coloring, her love of using color has always shone through.

As a Military Veteran, Wife and Mother of two, she has experienced long term anxiety & depression and continues to practice being mindful on a daily basis.

It was through therapy that she learnt to use her love for drawing and coloring to help relieve her symptoms of stress, anxiety & depression.

She found that through her coloring, a form of art therapy, it helped distract her mind's thought processes and had a relaxing and calming effect on her mind and body.

Nerine also discovered her flair for creating and designing mandalas and patterns and now enjoys designing her own coloring books.

It was from her personal and life experiences that she created the first of her series of Adult Coloring Books titled Mandalas for Mindfulness. Each coloring book has been designed with the focus of helping other Military Veterans, and Men and Women living with conditions such as stress, anxiety & depression.

Coloring has been found to be a mindful activity that can help reduce symptoms and stress levels, as well as having a calming effect on the mind and body.

She hopes you will enjoy coloring her coloring books as much as she has enjoyed creating them for you.

You can connect with Nerine and share your finished colored pages at:
www.facebook.com/ColorYourWayToHappy

You can also check out more of her adult coloring books in the series at: www.ColorYourWayToHappy.com and join her weekly newsletter to receive a FREE coloring book as well as new coloring pages, tips and helpful information on how to cope; living with stress, anxiety and depression.

Did you enjoy this coloring book?
If so, please take a moment and leave a review at:
www.ColorYourWayToHappy.com/Anxiety

MORE ADULT COLORING BOOKS BY NERINE MARTIN

Available on Amazon.com (search for Nerine Martin)
Also available from www.ColorYourWayToHappy.com

Share your colored pages from Nerine's books at:
www.facebook.com/ColorYourWayToHappy

The *Color Your Way To Happy* adult coloring book series,
offers you an escape from the daily pressures of life,
to a relaxing state of calm and mindfulness.

Grab your copy today and go 'Color Your Way To Happy'.

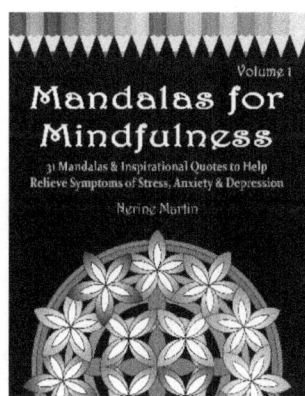
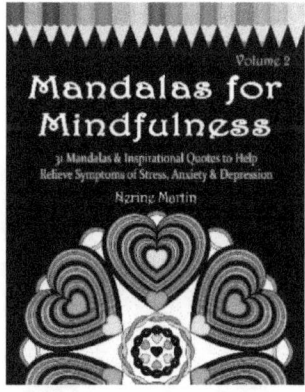
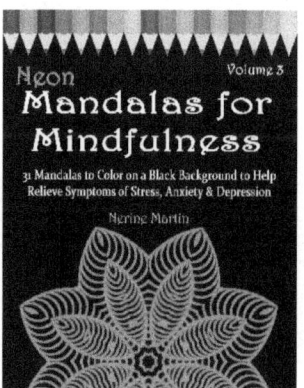
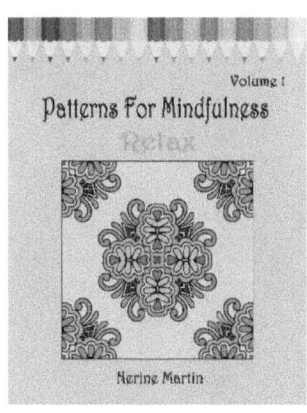
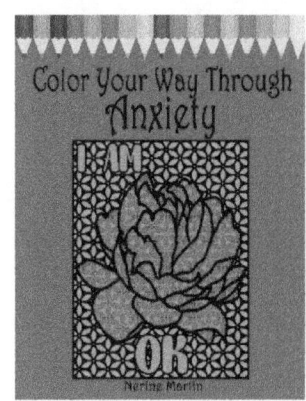
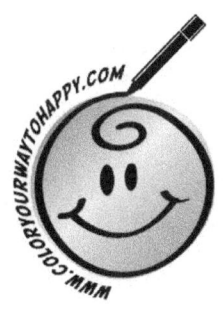